THE IMPACT OF GLOBALIZATION ON INFECTIOUS DISEASE EMERGENCE AND CONTROL

Exploring the Consequences and Opportunities

Workshop Summary

Stacey Knobler, Adel Mahmoud, Stanley Lemon
Editors

Forum on Microbial Threats

Board on Global Health

INSTITUTE OF MEDICINE
OF THE NATIONAL ACADEMIES

THE NATIONAL ACADEMIES PRESS
Washington, D.C.
www.nap.edu

THE NATIONAL ACADEMIES PRESS • 500 FIFTH STREET, N.W. • Washington, DC 20001

NOTICE: The project that is the subject of this report was approved by the Governing Board of the National Research Council, whose members are drawn from the councils of the National Academy of Sciences, the National Academy of Engineering, and the Institute of Medicine.

Support for this project was provided by the U.S. Department of Health and Human Services' National Institutes of Health, Centers for Disease Control and Prevention, and Food and Drug Administration; U.S. Agency for International Development; U.S. Department of Defense; U.S. Department of State; U.S. Department of Veterans Affairs; U.S. Department of Agriculture; American Society for Microbiology; Burroughs Wellcome Fund; Pfizer; GlaxoSmithKline; and the Merck Company Foundation. The views presented in this report are those of the editors and attributed authors and are not necessarily those of the funding agencies.

This report is based on the proceedings of a workshop that was sponsored by the Forum on Microbial Threats. It is prepared in the form of a workshop summary by and in the name of the editors, with the assistance of staff and consultants, as an individually authored document. Sections of the workshop summary not specifically attributed to an individual reflect the views of the editors and not those of the Forum on Microbial Threats. The content of those sections is based on the presentations and the discussions that took place during the workshop.

Library of Congress Cataloging-in-Publication Data

The impact of globalization on infectious disease emergence and control : exploring the consequences and opportunities : workshop summary / Stacey Knobler, Adel Mahmoud, Stanley Lemon, editors ; Forum on Microbial Threats ; Board on Global Health.
   p. ; cm.
   Includes bibliographical references.
   ISBN 0-309-10098-4 (pbk.)
   1.   Communicable diseases—Prevention—Congresses.   2. Communicable diseases—Prevention—Case studies—Congresses. I. Knobler, Stacey. II. Mahmoud, Adel A. F. III. Lemon, Stanley M. IV. Forum on Microbial Threats. V. Institute of Medicine (U.S.). Board on Global Health.
   [DNLM: 1. Communicable Disease Control—Congresses. 2. Communicable Diseases—transmission—Congresses. 3. Disease Outbreaks —prevention & control—Congresses. 4. Disease Transmission—prevention & control—Congresses. 5. Health Policy—Congresses. 6. International Cooperation—Congresses.   WA 110 I339 2006]
   RA643.I47 2006
   362.196'9—dc22
                                                                              2005036813

Additional copies of this report are available from the National Academies Press, 500 Fifth Street, N.W., Lockbox 285, Washington, DC 20055; (800) 624–6242 or (202) 334–3313 (in the Washington metropolitan area); Internet, http://www.nap.edu.

For more information about the Institute of Medicine, visit the IOM home page at: **www.iom.edu.**

The serpent has been a symbol of long life, healing, and knowledge among almost all cultures and religions since the beginning of recorded history. The serpent adopted as a logotype by the Institute of Medicine is a relief carving from ancient Greece, now held by the Staatliche Museen in Berlin.

COVER: The background for the cover of this workshop summary is a photograph of a batik designed and printed specifically for the Malaysian Society of Parasitology and Tropical Medicine. The print contains drawings of various parasites and insects; it is used with the kind permission of the Society.

"Knowing is not enough; we must apply. Willing is not enough; we must do."
—Goethe

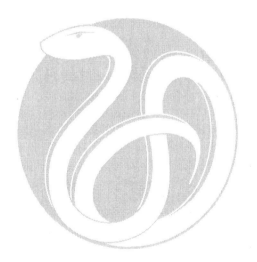

INSTITUTE OF MEDICINE
OF THE NATIONAL ACADEMIES

Advising the Nation. Improving Health.

THE NATIONAL ACADEMIES
Advisers to the Nation on Science, Engineering, and Medicine

The **National Academy of Sciences** is a private, nonprofit, self-perpetuating society of distinguished scholars engaged in scientific and engineering research, dedicated to the furtherance of science and technology and to their use for the general welfare. Upon the authority of the charter granted to it by the Congress in 1863, the Academy has a mandate that requires it to advise the federal government on scientific and technical matters. Dr. Ralph J. Cicerone is president of the National Academy of Sciences.

The **National Academy of Engineering** was established in 1964, under the charter of the National Academy of Sciences, as a parallel organization of outstanding engineers. It is autonomous in its administration and in the selection of its members, sharing with the National Academy of Sciences the responsibility for advising the federal government. The National Academy of Engineering also sponsors engineering programs aimed at meeting national needs, encourages education and research, and recognizes the superior achievements of engineers. Dr. Wm. A. Wulf is president of the National Academy of Engineering.

The **Institute of Medicine** was established in 1970 by the National Academy of Sciences to secure the services of eminent members of appropriate professions in the examination of policy matters pertaining to the health of the public. The Institute acts under the responsibility given to the National Academy of Sciences by its congressional charter to be an adviser to the federal government and, upon its own initiative, to identify issues of medical care, research, and education. Dr. Harvey V. Fineberg is president of the Institute of Medicine.

The **National Research Council** was organized by the National Academy of Sciences in 1916 to associate the broad community of science and technology with the Academy's purposes of furthering knowledge and advising the federal government. Functioning in accordance with general policies determined by the Academy, the Council has become the principal operating agency of both the National Academy of Sciences and the National Academy of Engineering in providing services to the government, the public, and the scientific and engineering communities. The Council is administered jointly by both Academies and the Institute of Medicine. Dr. Ralph J. Cicerone and Dr. Wm. A. Wulf are chair and vice chair, respectively, of the National Research Council.

www.national-academies.org

FORUM ON MICROBIAL THREATS

JANET SHOEMAKER, Director, Office of Public Affairs, American Society for Microbiology, Washington, D.C.

BRIAN STASKAWICZ, Professor, Department of Plant and Microbial Biology, University of California, Berkeley

TERENCE TAYLOR, President and Executive Director, International Institute for Strategic Studies, Washington, D.C.

Liaisons

ENRIQUETA BOND, President, Burroughs Wellcome Fund, Research Triangle Park, North Carolina

NANCY CARTER-FOSTER, Director, Program for Emerging Infections and HIV/AIDS, U.S. Department of State, Washington, D.C.

EDWARD McSWEEGAN, Program Officer, National Institute of Allergy and Infectious Diseases, National Institutes of Health, Bethesda, Maryland

Staff

EILEEN CHOFFNES, Director, Forum on Microbial Threats
STACEY KNOBLER, Former Director, Forum on Microbial Threats
THOMAS BURROUGHS, Science Writer
ELIZABETH KITCHENS, Research Associate
KIM LUNDBERG, Research Associate
KATHERINE McCLURE, Research Associate
KATE SKOCZDOPOLE, Senior Program Assistant

Reviewers

All presenters at the workshop have reviewed and approved their respective sections of this report for accuracy. In addition, this workshop summary has been reviewed in draft form by independent reviewers chosen for their diverse perspectives and technical expertise, in accordance with procedures approved by the National Research Council's Report Review Committee. The purpose of this independent review is to provide candid and critical comments that will assist the Institute of Medicine (IOM) in making the published workshop summary as sound as possible and to ensure that the workshop summary meets institutional standards. The review comments and draft manuscript remain confidential to protect the integrity of the deliberative process.

The Forum and IOM thank the following individuals for their participation in the review process:

Nick Drager, Department of Ethics, Trade, Human Rights and Law World Health Organization, Geneva, Switzerland.

Johannes Sommerfeld, Special Programme for Research and Training in Tropical Diseases (TDR) World Health Organization, Geneva, Switzerland.

Mary Wilson, Harvard University, Boston, Massachusetts

The review of this report was overseen by **Melvin Worth, M.D.,** Scholar-in-Residence, National Academies, who was responsible for making certain that an independent examination of this report was carried out in accordance with institutional procedures and that all review comments were carefully considered. Responsibility for the final content of this report rests entirely with the editors and the institution.

Preface

The Forum on Emerging Infections was created in 1996 in response to a request from the Centers for Disease Control and Prevention and the National Institutes of Health. The goal of the Forum is to provide structured opportunities for representatives from academia, industry, professional and interest groups, and government[1] to examine and discuss scientific and policy issues that are of shared interest and that are specifically related to research and prevention, detection, and management of infectious diseases. In accomplishing this task, the Forum provides the opportunity to foster the exchange of information and ideas, identify areas in need of greater attention, clarify policy issues by enhancing knowledge and identifying points of agreement, and inform decision makers about science and policy issues. The Forum seeks to illuminate issues rather than resolve them directly; hence, it does not provide advice or recommendations on any specific policy initiative pending before any agency or organization. Its strengths are the diversity of its membership and the contributions of individual members expressed throughout the activities of the Forum. In September of 2003 the Forum changed its name to the Forum on Microbial Threats.

---

[1]Representatives of federal agencies serve in an ex officio capacity. An ex officio member of a group is one who is a member automatically by virtue of holding a particular office or membership in another body.

ABOUT THE WORKSHOP

We live in a time of unprecedented human movement and interaction. As transborder mobility of humans, animals, food, and feed products increases, so does the threat of the spread of infectious disease. While new global markets have created economic opportunities and growth, the benefits have not been equally distributed, and the risks—especially the health risks—of our increasingly interconnected and fast-paced world continue to grow. Although the burden is greatest for the developing world, infectious diseases are a growing threat to all nations.

The resurgence of malaria is a dramatic example of the effects of globalization on disease trends. Twenty years ago, more than 80 percent of the world's population lived in malaria-free or controlled areas. But today, malaria is the most prevalent vectorborne disease, with more than 40 percent of the world's population living in endemic areas. Furthermore, with increased air travel and human movement, imported malaria is on the rise in Europe and North America. The AIDS pandemic and the global spread of the annual influenza virus further illustrate how vulnerable even industrialized nations are to unexpected outbreaks and the spread of infectious disease in today's globalized society.

However, the same globalizing forces that create such rampant opportunity for pathogens also can provide mechanisms for innovative, global efforts to control infectious diseases. A new network of international public health partners is emerging. Multinational partnerships are contributing to the increased availability of drugs and vaccines, the development of health care infrastructures in developing countries, and better public health education programs worldwide. The global proliferation of technology and information has the potential to improve the identification, surveillance, containment, and treatment of disease in both developed and developing countries. Growing international cooperation may lead to more robust and transparent reporting regarding disease outbreaks and control efforts. Distance learning, training, and research exchange programs are creating improved access for scientific and medical professionals.

On April 16 and 17, 2002, the Forum on Emerging Infections held a working group discussion on the influence of globalization on the emergence and control of infectious diseases. Through invited presentations and participant discussion, the workshop explored the impact of increasingly integrated trade, economic development, human movement, and cultural exchange on patterns of disease emergence; identified opportunities for countering the effects of globalization on infectious diseases; examined the scientific evidence supporting current and potential global strategies; and considered newly available response methods and tools available for use by private industry, public health agencies, regulatory agencies, policy makers, and academic researchers. During the last session of the workshop, Forum members, panel discussants, and the audience commented on issues and next steps that they consider priority areas for action.

ORGANIZATION OF WORKSHOP SUMMARY

This workshop summary was prepared for the Forum membership in the name of the editors, with the assistance of staff and consultants. The sections of this summary that are not specifically attributed to an individual reflect the views of the editors exclusively—they do not reflect the views of the Institute of Medicine (IOM) or of the organizations that sponsor the Forum on Microbial Threats. The contents of the unattributed sections are based on the presentations and discussions that took place during the workshop.

The globalization workshop functioned as a venue for dialogue among representatives from many sectors about their beliefs on subjects that may merit further attention. The reader should be aware that the material presented here reflects the views and opinions of those participating in the workshop and not the deliberations of a formally constituted IOM study committee. Moreover, these proceedings summarize only what participants stated in the workshop and are not intended to be an exhaustive exploration of the subject matter.

This summary is organized as a topic-by-topic description of the presentations and discussions from the workshop. The purpose is to present lessons from relevant experience, delineate a range of pivotal issues and their respective problems, and put forth some potential responses as described by the workshop participants. The Summary and Assessment discusses the core messages that emerged from the working group discussions. Chapter 1 summarizes the presentations and discussions related to the increasing cross-border and cross-continental movements of people, products, pathogens, and power, and how these affect the emergence and spread of infectious diseases. Chapter 2 provides a summary of the presentations and discussions that revolved around the changing global landscape and how this could exacerbate the emergence and global spread of infectious diseases. Chapter 3 focuses on the opportunities and obstacles surrounding the global application of knowledge, tools, and technology that result from increasing globalization. Chapter 4 summarizes the means by which sovereign states and nations must adopt a global public health mind-set and develop a new organizational framework to maximize the opportunities and overcome the challenges created by globalization and build the necessary capacity to respond effectively to emerging infectious disease threats.

ACKNOWLEDGMENTS

The Forum on Microbial Threats and IOM wish to express their warmest appreciation to the individuals and organizations who gave valuable time to provide information and advice to the Forum through participation in the workshop (see Appendix A for a list of speakers).

The Forum is indebted to the IOM staff who contributed during the course of the workshop and to the production of this workshop summary. On behalf of the Forum, we gratefully acknowledge the efforts led by Stacey Knobler, director of the Forum, and Leslie Pray, technical consultant, who dedicated much effort and time to developing the workshop agenda, and thank them for their thoughtful and insightful approach and skill in translating the workshop proceedings and discussion into this summary.

Finally, the Forum also thanks sponsors that supported this activity. Financial support for this project was provided by the U.S. Department of Health and Human Services' National Institutes of Health, Centers for Disease Control and Prevention, and Food and Drug Administration; U.S. Department of Defense; U.S. Department of State; U.S. Department of Veterans Affairs; U.S. Department of Agriculture; American Society for Microbiology; Burroughs Wellcome Fund; Pfizer; GlaxoSmithKline; and the Merck Company Foundation. The views presented in this workshop summary are those of the editors and workshop participants and are not necessarily those of the funding organizations.

Adel Mahmoud, Chair
Stanley Lemon, Vice-Chair
Forum on Microbial Threats

Contents

xv

THE IMPACT OF GLOBALIZATION ON INFECTIOUS DISEASE EMERGENCE AND CONTROL

Summary and Assessment

The cold war era has passed. The fall of the Berlin Wall in 1989 marked the beginning of the disappearance of old borders and a new global era of unparalleled human movement and interaction. Although the new global arena has created economic opportunities and growth, the benefits have not been equally distributed, and the risks—especially the health risks—of this increasingly interconnected and fast-paced world continue to grow. As people, products, food, and capital travel the world in unprecedented numbers and at historic speeds, so, too, do the myriad of disease-causing microorganisms. The worldwide resurgence of dengue fever, the introduction of West Nile virus into New York City in 1999, the rapid spread of human immunodeficiency virus (HIV) infection in Russia, and the global spread of multidrug-resistant tuberculosis (TB) are but a few examples of the profound effects of globalizing forces on the emergence, distribution, and spread of infectious diseases. No nation is immune to the growing global threat that can be posed by an isolated outbreak of infectious disease in a seemingly remote part of the world. Today, whether carried by an unknowing traveler or an opportunistic vector, human pathogens can rapidly arrive anywhere in the world.

At the same time, the very interdependency and connectedness that create such opportunities for the global spread of pathogens also offer mechanisms for innovative, multinational efforts to address the threat. A growing network of such efforts, combined with the global proliferation of technology and information, continues to strengthen the global public health capacity to prevent and control the spread of emerging and reemerging

1

infectious diseases. One participant in the Workshop on the Impact of Globalization on Infectious Disease Emergence and Control described the situation thus: just as the globalization of infectious diseases is characterized by a transformation of separate entities into a unified epidemiological system, disease control capacity in one part of the globe can readily be deployed to fight diseases in other parts of the world.

Workshop participants discussed the impacts of increasingly integrated trade, economic development, human movement, and cultural exchange on patterns of disease emergence and reemergence; identified opportunities for countering those impacts; examined the scientific evidence supporting current and potential global strategies; and considered new response methods and tools available for use by private industry, public health agencies, regulatory agencies, policy makers, and academic researchers. Participants included experts from the international community, industry, academia, the public health community, and government; invited international participants included key representatives from the Americas, the European Union, and Russia. Detailed summaries of the workshop's formal presentations and roundtable discussions are presented in Chapters 1 through 4 of this report.

At one point during the workshop, a call was made to heed the danger of equating globalization with Americanization, as an international point of view is crucial to a true understanding of the issues. Participants were also asked to strike a balance between what could be perceived as the negative aspects of globalization and its humanizing and empowering potential. As one participant explained, to examine the globalization of emerging infectious disease, one must address a more general tension that characterizes any globalization phenomenon: that between globalization as opportunity, the view taken by Friedman (2000) in *The Lexus and the Olive Tree*, and as something that is frightening and potentially dangerous, the perspective taken in the more radical social scientific literature (see Appendix A). As another participant put it, while examining the responses needed to meet this Malthusian challenge, one concludes that the solutions may be unearthed from the problem.

THE PAST, PRESENT, AND FUTURE OF THE
GLOBALIZATION OF INFECTIOUS DISEASE

Globalization is by no means a new phenomenon; transcontinental trade and the movement of people date back at least 2,000 years, to the era of the ancient Silk Road trade route. The global spread of infectious disease has followed a parallel course. Indeed, the emergence and spread of infectious disease are, in a sense, the epitome of globalization. By Roman times, world trade routes had effectively joined Europe, Asia, and North America into one giant breeding ground for microbes. Millions of Roman citizens were killed between 165 and 180 AD when smallpox finally reached Rome during the Plague of Antoninus. Three centuries later, the bubonic plague hit Europe for the first time (542–543 AD) as the Plague of Justinian. It returned in full force as the Black Death in the fourteenth century, when a new route for overland trade with China provided rapid transit for flea-infested furs from plague-ridden Central Asia.

Even before the development of world trade routes, however, human pathogens had experienced two major bonanzas. First, when people lived as hunter-gatherers, they were constantly on the move, making it difficult for microbes to keep up with their human hosts. Once people started living as farmers, they began residing in larger numbers in the same place—and were in daily contact with their accumulating feces—for extended periods of time. Second, the advent of cities brought even larger numbers of people together under even worse sanitary conditions. In the Middle Ages, when people threw human waste out their windows in England, they were said to be "blessing the passerby."

Now, two millennia later, human pathogens are experiencing yet another bonanza from a new era of globalization characterized by faster travel over greater distances and worldwide trade. Although some experts mark the fall of the Berlin Wall as the beginning of this new era, others argue that it is not so new. Even a hundred years ago, at the turn of the nineteenth century, the tremendous impact of increased trade and travel on infectious disease was evident in the emergence of plague epidemics in numerous port cities around the world. As Echenberg (2002) notes, plague epidemics in colonial African cities were closely tied to the increased communication, travel, and trade that accompanied the advent of the steamship. The economic and social impacts of these epidemics were profound. In Johannesburg, in what is now South Africa, the occurrence of plague led to the relocation of black residents in an effort to remove what the white colonists believed was the source of the disease. At about the same time, the influenza pandemic killed many millions of people worldwide.

Thus the current era of globalization is more properly viewed as an intensification of trends that have occurred throughout history. Never before have so many people moved so quickly throughout the world, whether by choice or force. Never before has the population density been higher, with more people living in urban areas. Never before have food, animals, commodities, and capital been transported so freely and quickly across political boundaries. And never before have pathogens had such ample opportunity to hitch global rides on airplanes, people, and products.

The future of globalization is still in the making. Despite the successful attempts of the developed world during the course of the last century to control many infectious diseases and even to eradicate some deadly afflic-

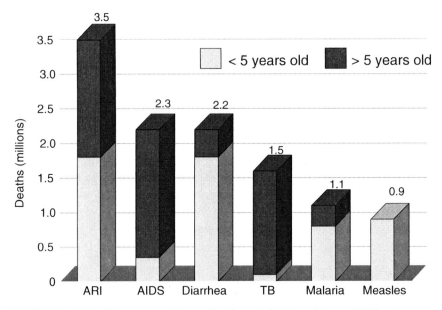

FIGURE S-1 Leading causes of mortality from infectious disease, 2000 estimates.
SOURCE: Klaucke (2002).

tions, 13 million people worldwide still die from such diseases every year (see Figure S-1).

Although the burden is greatest for the developing world, infectious diseases are a growing threat to all nations. The problem is compounded by the emergence of new diseases, such as severe acute respiratory syndrome (SARS),[1] that occur unexpectedly and require urgent interventions (see Figures S-2a and S-2b).

The uncertainties of what can and will happen posed challenges to the workshop participants as they discussed the issues. At the same time, their collective wisdom presented opportunities to establish a framework for progress. The growing threat of the emergence, reemergence, and rapid global spread of infectious disease calls for a new, global paradigm of participation by the public health community. The need for collaboration has never been greater. Long-term, multinational training and partnerships among government, health care, financial, and other institutions are vital to building the global public health capacity necessary to address the threat posed worldwide by even an isolated incident of an infectious disease. The

---

[1]Although SARS did not emerge until after this workshop was held, it is mentioned here as a timely example.

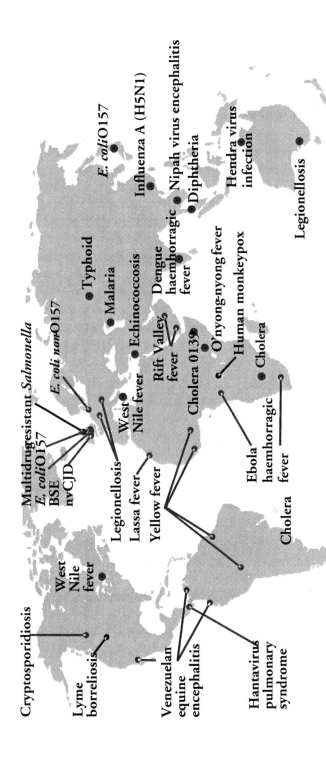

FIGURE S-2a   Emerging and reemerging diseases, 1996–2001.
SOURCE: Klaucke (2002).

6

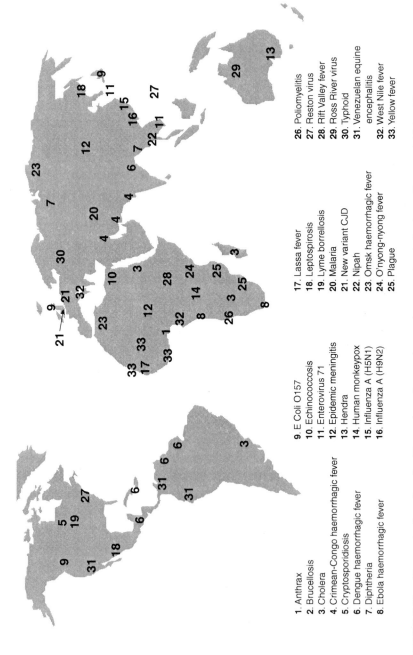

1. Anthrax
2. Brucellosis
3. Cholera
4. Crimean-Congo haemorrhagic fever
5. Cryptosporidiosis
6. Dengue haemorrhagic fever
7. Diphtheria
8. Ebola haemorrhagic fever

9. E Coli O157
10. Echinococcosis
11. Enterovirus 71
12. Epidemic meningitis
13. Hendra
14. Human monkeypox
15. Influenza A (H5N1)
16. Influenza A (H9N2)

17. Lassa fever
18. Leptospirosis
19. Lyme borrelliosis
20. Malaria
21. New variant CJD
22. Nipah
23. Omsk haemorrhagic fever
24. O'nyong-nyong fever
25. Plague

26. Poliomyelitis
27. Reston virus
28. Rift Valley fever
29. Ross River virus
30. Typhoid
31. Venezuelan equine encephalitis
32. West Nile fever
33. Yellow fever

FIGURE S-2b Unexpected outbreaks: Examples of emerging and reemerging infectious diseases, 1994–1999. SOURCE: WHO (1999).

full and equal participation of partners in the developing world will be critical to this effort.

What exactly does such a collaborative, international framework entail? What opportunities does globalization afford to support the effort? How can these new global tools be used to their maximum advantage? What obstacles must be overcome? These are some of the many questions deliberated by the workshop participants, as summarized in this report.

Chapters 1 and 2 describe how globalizing forces have affected the prevention and control of infectious disease. The topics discussed range from the impact of the international flow of capital on emerging infectious diseases to the opportunities provided by the new, unprecedented influx of spending on defense against bioterrorism. Chapter 3 describes a variety of new opportunities for enhancing infectious disease control, such as global surveillance capabilities and the changing nature of transnational public health training programs. Chapter 4 summarizes some key components of the new global public health framework: the role of public–private partnerships, the role of international law, and the importance of a social science perspective for understanding and studying emerging infectious diseases. Finally, the appendices to this report consist of the workshop agenda and papers contributed by David Fidler, Jonathan Mayer, and Andrey Demin.

A WORLD IN MOTION

As the human immunodeficiency virus (HIV) disease pandemic surely should have taught us, in the context of infectious diseases, there is nowhere in the world from which we are remote and no one from whom we are disconnected.

— IOM, 1992

Over the past two centuries, the average distance and speed of human travel have increased a thousand-fold, but incubation times for infectious diseases have remained the same. What historically may have been only a small, localized outbreak can now develop in a matter of days into a large, worldwide epidemic. Not only have the speed and distance of human travel accelerated and expanded, but unprecedented numbers of people are also on the move. Thirty years ago there were only about 200 million international tourist arrivals annually, compared with an expected 900 million or more by 2010. The global spread of HIV/AIDS is only one, albeit the most devastating, example of the impact of this tremendous human mobility on infectious disease.

Tourists are not the only people taking advantage of open borders and international travel opportunities. Each year millions of people leave their homes, either temporarily or permanently, in search of work or an improved quality of life, and millions more are forcibly displaced by war. These migrant populations, especially refugees, are among the most vulnerable to emerging infectious diseases. In many developed countries, the emergence and reemergence of infectious diseases, such as multidrug-resistant TB, are frequently linked to the massive influx of immigrants from poor countries with a higher prevalence of such diseases. The situation is expected to worsen in the future as the world population grows, demographic and economic gaps between the developed and developing worlds deepen, and greater numbers of people either are forcibly displaced or leave their homes by choice in search of a better life.

Although increased human mobility may be the most obvious manifestation of globalization, it is by no means the most important. As several workshop participants noted, the global spread of capitalism and the free market is the main driving force behind the current era of globalization. Much discussion at the workshop thus focused on the rapidly changing nature of the global marketplace; the ease with which food, commodities, capital, and economic and political decision-making powers are being passed around the world; and the important implications of these changes for infectious disease emergence and control.

The same advances in transportation technology that facilitate global travel by humans also allow the rapid transcontinental movement of infectious disease vectors. It has been hypothesized, for example, that the vehicle for the introduction of West Nile virus into the United States in 1999, the first occurrence of this disease in the western hemisphere, was an airplane carrying an infected mosquito vector (Cetron, 2002). That mosquito vectors can hitch rides in the wheel wells of airplanes is well known. Controversial evidence also suggests that global warming, much of which is generated by human trade-related activities, may be leading to an increase in the geographic expansion and distribution of vectors.

Historically, most food has been produced and consumed locally. Over the last two decades, however, as consumer demand and expectations have increased and as food production and processing activities have become more geographically fragmented (e.g., foods produced in one locale being processed elsewhere), the epidemiology of foodborne disease has changed significantly. More recently, changes in international trade law, including the establishment of the World Trade Organization (WTO) in 1995, have altered even more dramatically the ways in which all products, food and others, are bought and sold. For example, before the establishment of WTO in 1995, trade in animals and animal products was conducted according to a policy of zero risk. Now, imported products are treated no less favorably than domestic products, at least with regard to animal health restrictions. The experience of bovine spongiform encephalopathy in the United Kingdom and Europe illustrates the tremendous risk that accompanies the seemingly unlimited growth and opportunity offered by new international trade regulations enforced by WTO.

It is cause for alarm that many countries do not have comprehensive food safety programs integrated into their public health strategies. The problem is not limited to the developing world or to food products imported from those nations. Outbreaks of foodborne illness have revealed several inadequacies in food safety regulation capabilities even in the United States. The free flow of food also raises serious concerns about the global spread of antibiotic resistance associated with the consumption of antibiotic-fed food animals.

Finally, although the use of the term "globalization" in the health sciences literature generally refers to growing global interdependency, particularly as manifested by increased international travel, the phenomenon of globalization encompasses much more. It also refers to the changing nature of the world's global political economy, the development of a truly global marketplace, and the power relationships embedded within this new economy. In fact, given that the spread of capitalism and the free market is the main driving force behind globalization, the health sciences community might benefit from examining the ways in which this movement of capital affects emerging infectious diseases. An excellent demonstration of this point is the use of foreign capital to fund dam construction and other similar environmental modification projects, which almost always alter, either directly or indirectly, local vector ecologies and human–pathogen interactions. For example, not only is construction of the Three Gorges Dam on the Yangtze River in China altering the potential for the transmission of schistosomiasis and other diseases by disrupting local vector ecologies, but it is also increasing the risk of transmission even further by forcing people to leave their homes and live in highly concentrated areas. In light of the damaging effects of many projects on their local and regional environments and public health, workshop participants suggested that perhaps current economic models need to be reexamined, and that the potential (and costly) public health ramifications of investment decisions need somehow to be incorporated into those models.

EXAMINING THE CONSEQUENCES

As the public health ramifications of dam construction and other environmental modification projects illustrate, the growing international market and the increased mobility of the global population have already and will continue to play a central role in shaping the global infectious disease landscape, both literally and figuratively. Other global developments discussed at the workshop have important public health implications as well, including globally fueled armed conflicts and the massive displacement of people, the inability to monitor and provide adequate health care to the continually growing numbers of mobile people displaced because of war or other reasons, the incapacity to monitor foodborne and trade-related infectious disease risks worldwide, and the growing actual and perceived threats of bioterrorism. These developments have at least one thing in common: if left unchecked, they could have profound and potentially devastating consequences for global public health.

Some argue that as the global economy improves, the living conditions of poor populations will also improve. As one participant suggested, however, this is not necessarily true. Poor countries of the world are still poor, violence is increasing, and the same diseases still exist. As information becomes easier to access in even the remotest corners of the world, everyone will know how everyone else is living and under what circumstances. Greater numbers of people will leave their homes in search of work and an improved quality of life, and greater numbers of people will be forcibly displaced. As the world population continues to grow, as urban areas in the developing world continue to expand and further strain their already resource-limited governments, and as the global marketplace continues to hone the already sharp demarcation in wealth—and health—that exists between rich and poor countries, the ensuing social unrest and loss of state control will likely fuel even more communal conflict, forced migration, and terrorism.

Unless the public health infrastructure is modified to accommodate the health care needs of mobile populations and unless the capacity to monitor mobile populations is strengthened, both pre- and postarrival, the United States and other developed countries will be unable to handle the massive influx of immigrant and refugee populations. One participant described the surveillance of mobile populations as a "new but necessary idea." The global spread of TB, particularly multidrug-resistant TB, illustrates what can result from the failure to monitor and provide health care for mobile populations. The gap in the prevalence of TB between U.S.-born and foreign-born U.S. residents is already huge; according to the Centers for Disease Control and Prevention, foreign-born residents accounted for 46 percent of new cases of TB in the United States in 2000 (CDC, 2002). Other developed countries are experiencing the same phenomenon; for example, according to a 1998 study, 92 percent of all multidrug-resistant TB cases in Canada were imported (Grondin, 2002). Not only are migrants and refugees more likely than the general population to become infected, but they also put others at risk.

Standards are therefore needed for monitoring the health of mobile populations. While such standards are necessary, however, they will not be sufficient. Unless their underlying causes are addressed, armed conflict and the threat of terrorism will continue to plague the world, drive mass migra-

---

Box S-1
Cyclosporiasis Outbreaks in California

In a retrospective study, Mohle-Boetani and colleagues (2000) analyzed a number of factors that contributed to the recognition of cyclosporiasis during eight months of outbreaks in California in the spring of 1997. The authors interviewed index patients with the disease and reviewed the proportion of cases detected because of enhanced laboratory surveillance. Diagnosis of cyclosporiasis requires special testing not done with standard ova and parasite methods. Six of the eight index cases were diagnosed more than two weeks after onset of symptoms. In six of the eight cases, stool testing was done after patients brought information to their physicians and requested the tests. The information came from Internet searches and from newspapers and other media coverage. In one instance, a physician was prompted by a television report to test for cyclosporiasis.

Multiple communication channels link physicians and patients and educate both. This study shows how knowledge derived from websites and the media led to the diagnosis of a disease previously unknown to many clinicians. Enhanced laboratory surveillance also contributed to detection of the parasite.

SOURCE: Mohle-Boetani et al. (2000).

---

tion, and increase the risk of the emergence and spread of infectious disease. In the case of wars, almost all of which involve the use of small arms, workshop participants cited limiting the availability of such arms as an example of a tangible step that could be taken, given that the legal small arms trade is amenable to modification through U.S. policy (Leaning, 2002).

As with the monitoring of mobile populations, unless the capacity to monitor the global transport of foodborne and trade-related vectorborne infectious diseases is improved, such diseases will continue to pose serious public health risks. Although some argue that the risk of imported foodborne disease is relatively low—at least in the United States and in comparison with the risk of domestically derived foodborne disease—others argue that the surprisingly low incidence of the former reflects more a lack of surveillance than a lack of disease. The 1996–1998 outbreaks of *cyclosporiasis* in North America, caused by contaminated raspberries imported from Guatemala (see Box S-1), may not be as isolated an incident as one might think. One of the reasons this outbreak received so much attention was the scientific excitement surrounding the relatively newly discovered pathogenic culprit. Yet even if foodborne outbreaks caused by imported products are uncommon, the potential for such outbreaks is increasing. Although WTO, the World Health Organization (WHO), the Asia-Pacific Economic Cooperation (APEC), and a handful of other regional organizations have recently attempted to improve surveillance for foodborne and trade-related infectious diseases, this is still a somewhat underappreciated need.

Finally, one of the most prominent features of the new global landscape is the increased threat of bioterrorism. As one participant put it, today we are standing at the crossroads of two historical trajectories: one stemming from a day in 1453 when Constantinople fell to the Turks after centuries of conflict between the Christian West and the Muslim East, an event that signified the end of the Middle Ages and the beginning of the Renaissance; the other stemming from an event that occurred nearly 500 years later, when the British scientific journal *Nature* published an article by two young scientists, James Watson and Frances Crick, reporting the discovery of the DNA double helix. Thus, as the world enters the twenty-first century, society is simultaneously witnessing the reemergence of conflict between western and eastern cultures, the denouement of the age of physics, and the ascendance of the age of biology. The result is the convergence of global terrorism and the widespread availability of molecular biology techniques. At the heart of this collision is the use of infectious disease as a weapon.

The threat of increased bioterrorism was made real by the terrorist attacks of September 11, 2001, and the subsequent mailing of letters laden with anthrax spores in October 2001. The challenges faced by international health programs have increased as a result. The current Bush Administration has responded with a 319 percent increase in spending on defense against bioterrorism—to $5.9 billion for fiscal year 2003. The funds will be used to improve detection and surveillance systems, strengthen medical capabilities, improve planning and coordination, foster research, expand training exercises and communication strategies, and address policies that create bureaucratic barriers to strengthening the U.S. capacity to address bioterrorism. The promised funding will potentially provide many new opportunities to strengthen the U.S. public health capacity to address multiple emerging infectious disease threats, both domestically and worldwide. This unprecedented level of funding offers a rare chance to make a difference in the surveillance and prevention of infectious diseases, although workshop participants expressed several concerns regarding the use and the sustainability of this funding.

OPPORTUNITIES AND OBSTACLES

The recent funding for biodefense initiatives is but one example of the many benefits of the globalization of efforts to combat microbial threats. Other benefits and advances include the growth and changing nature of training and research partnerships between developed and developing countries, the development of new treatments and vaccines that could potentially save millions of lives, and advances in information technology.

Despite a century of European involvement and decades of U.S. involvement in tropical medicine and infectious disease research and training programs, only recently have partnerships between developed and developing countries (also termed North–South partnerships) evolved into the type of egalitarian, bidirectional arrangement required for the global control of infectious disease. Most such programs, such as that of the Liverpool School of Tropical Medicine, founded in Liverpool, England, in 1898, were originally designed to develop Northern capacity and expertise in tropical medicine. However, to develop the global public health capacity needed to respond rapidly and effectively to an unexpected pandemic, whether introduced naturally or intentionally, more resources and focus must be directed toward strengthening the public health capacity of the developing world.

Several participants cited the Peru-based Gorgas Course in Clinical Tropical Medicine, a collaborative effort between the University of Alabama and the Instituto de Medicina Tropical "Alexander von Humboldt," as an example of the kind of program that is needed. This collaboration empowers its Southern participants in a way that lays the groundwork for building a sustainable intellectual and public health capacity in that developing nation. The Fogarty International Center of the National Institutes of Health is undertaking similar efforts by planning and implementing a range of training programs overseas.

The need to strengthen the public health capacity in the developing world should not, however, detract from the still urgent need to incorporate public health education and training into the curricula of U.S. medical and veterinary schools. A number of recent microbial threats have been zoonotic. To address these and other future threats effectively, links need to be established between medical and veterinary schools. Human and animal health issues must be addressed in a coordinated manner if the public health workforce is to be trained to combat zoonotic diseases. Moreover, many practicing physicians in developed nations have never seen a case of measles, let alone malaria. Thus, transnational programs should continue to serve the original goal of strengthening the public health capacity in the North as well. After all, there is much to be learned in and from the developing world.

Peru has a long and rich history of experience with infectious diseases. For example, Peruvian mummies have yielded evidence that the first known TB epidemic occurred in that country nearly 2,000 years ago. Several hundred years ago, Spaniards introduced smallpox into Peru when they first landed on the shores of the Americas (Peru, in turn, sent syphilis back to sixteenth-century Europe, where Spanish troops spread the epidemic throughout the continent). In the last 25 years, one-third of all new infectious diseases described in the published literature have been discovered in Latin America. And the upwelling of the cold deep water off the coast of Peru, a decidedly local phenomenon, has become a worldwide problem in the form of the El Niño[2] Southern Oscillation, which in turn has had a significant effect on the ecology and public health–related consequences of infectious diseases worldwide.

North-south training partnerships are but one example of the type of multinational collaboration that the increasing interconnectedness of the world not only allows but demands. Workshop participants also cited the vital source of expertise and knowledge of infectious diseases represented by scientists from the former Soviet Union and the potential role Russia could play in transnational public health education and training.

Russia has been participating in other international efforts to prevent and control the emergence and reemergence of infectious diseases. Leading the way is the State Research Center of Virology and Biotechnology Vector (SRC VB Vector) in Koltsovo. Despite the achievements of SCR VB Vector, however, an enormous amount of work remains to be done to strengthen Russia's public health capacity. The country is experiencing the emergence and reemergence of multiple infectious disease agents, from hepatitis A virus to HIV and is on the verge of experiencing major epidemics. This crisis has been attributed to the tremendous economic, social, and public health fallout from the dissolution of the former Soviet Union. The pieces have yet to come back together again, and Russian leaders are urgently in need of a new public health paradigm.

As the situation in Russia demonstrates, taking full advantage of new global opportunities does not necessarily come easily. Antiretroviral agents, for example, have more than proven their public health worth in the United States and other developed countries for the treatment of HIV and other infections. However, sub-Saharan Africa—the region of the world worst affected by HIV/AIDS—and other resource-constrained settings are in urgent need of a way to scale up the delivery of antiretroviral therapy. It would be neither prudent nor practical to apply the U.S. model of the introduction and dissemination of antiretroviral agents. HIV infections resistant to antiretroviral agents have already become a serious problem in the United States, in part because of premature introduction of the drugs; if

---

[2]El Niño is a warming of the surface waters of the tropical Pacific that occurs every 3–5 years, temporarily affecting weather worldwide. The irregular cycling back and forth between warm and cold phases of the El Niño Southern Oscillation cycle in the equatorial Pacific results from a complex interplay between the strength of surface winds that blow westward along the equator and subsurface currents and temperatures. El Niño events are marked by higher-than-average pressure over the western Pacific and lower-than-average pressure over the eastern Pacific.

resistance to these agents emerges in Africa, it is likely that no amount of money or political will be able to stem the resulting crisis.

In addition, although vaccines have more than earned their reputation as one of the greatest public health tools in history, their utility in many developing countries is limited by weak or nonexistent public health infrastructures and a lack of resources. Despite the early successes of the Global Alliance for Vaccines and Immunization—formed in 2000 in response to the growing gap in levels of vaccine usage between developed and developing countries—numerous impediments to accelerating the global deployment of the available vaccines remain. For example, the limitations imposed by local conditions must be accounted for if new public health measures are to be implemented and new technologies transferred. Also, in the rush to achieve desirable short-term outcomes, local programs tend to be scaled up rapidly. The sudden infusion of billions of dollars into these systems, however, raises the question of how quickly this money can be spent wisely. Too often, hasty decisions have detrimental long-term consequences, and the cure ends up being worse than the problem.

Drug and vaccine delivery is only half of the problem. Equally urgent is the need to redress the imbalance between drug research and development efforts directed toward developed and developing nations. As one participant noted, although pharmaceutical companies have produced more than 2,000 new compounds over the last decade, only six of these are for the treatment of tropical diseases. As the global economy becomes even more interconnected, this will likely become an extremely difficult challenge to overcome.

Global surveillance is another example of a tool that holds tremendous promise but still faces many difficult political, scientific, and coordination challenges. Many countries fail to report local outbreaks in an effort to avoid potentially huge negative economic and political repercussions, such as trade sanctions and travel advisories. For several reasons, international reactions to public reports of infectious disease outbreaks typically far exceed what is warranted by the actual situation and public health risks. Even regional surveillance can be difficult to achieve, as the efforts in the Caribbean demonstrate (Corber, 2002).

A novel but for the most part untested idea introduced during the workshop was the establishment of a global public health bank for the storage and distribution of limited resources that might otherwise not be used to their maximum advantage. It was suggested that this program could be managed by a global health broker and would enable resources to be shared across borders (Timpieri, 2002).

Finally, most would agree that the Internet offers obvious and tremendous potential for infectious disease surveillance, prevention, and control. Never before have information and data been so easy to access and share.

The Global Outbreak Alert and Response Network (http://www.who.int/csr/outbreaknetwork/en/) and the Global Atlas of Infectious Diseases (http://www.whqathena.who.int/globalatlas/) are but two examples of how the Internet and other advances in information technology are being exploited in the fight against infectious diseases.

FRAMEWORK FOR PROGRESS

Recent large increases in spending on international health—for example, through the Global Fund to Fight AIDS, Tuberculosis, and Malaria and President Bush's recently proposed Millennium Challenge Account—reflect growing awareness and appreciation of the importance of global health. A number of factors account for these changing perceptions. First and foremost, support for international health efforts is no longer perceived as a costly charity endeavor; rather, it has become a cost-effective way of doing business. Even a century ago, millionaire ship owner Sir Alfred Lewis Jones founded the Liverpool School of Tropical Medicine, which sponsored 32 expeditions to the tropics between 1989 and 1913. Jones and other members of the Liverpool, England, business community recognized the wisdom of investing in the study of tropical diseases given that employee illnesses and deaths from malaria abroad led to reduced productivity and increased health expenditures at home.

Not only is poor public health bad for business, but it also threatens international political stability and U.S. national security. For example, at the same time that high HIV infection rates in sub-Saharan Africa limit the potential for international trade partnerships, they threaten the political and social stability of the entire region, thus posing a significant national security risk to the United States. The situation is exacerbated when armed forces are hit by high HIV infection rates, weakening military and peace-keeping capacities.

Despite increased funding and dramatic changes in the general perception of international health, several participants agreed that strengthening the global capacity to prevent and control the emergence and spread of infectious diseases will require even more money and newer approaches. Others emphasized the importance of recognizing the difference between the need for more money and the need to spend the available money more wisely. Without a strong infrastructure and knowledge base in place, large influxes of money are often wasted. It is crucial, therefore, that international systems and local agencies have the capacity to program significant amounts of money effectively. On the other hand, the tremendous amount of resources needed to address the most pressing global health problems, such as the HIV/AIDS pandemic and the global spread of drug-resistant malaria, cannot and should not be underestimated.

Participants identified four key components of a newer approach to infectious disease control:

- A global mind-set,
- Long-term collaborations, particularly public–private partnerships, among states, interstate and regional organizations, nongovernmental organizations, multinational corporations, and various other nonstate actors,
- Larger, more flexible financial consortiums, such as the Global Fund to Fight AIDS, Tuberculosis, and Malaria, and
- The concept of public goods, especially with regard to product development and the dissemination of knowledge.

With regard to the need for a global mind-set, the colors of the geopolitical map in no way reflect what is going on epidemiologically. A rational approach to infectious disease control must be based on science, not political boundaries. At the same time, however, public health agencies are generally constrained by the reality that they operate according to politically defined organizational structures. India, for example, has more than 50 different zones, each with its unique epidemiological conditions, yet the country is treated by WHO as a single unit or member state (Miller, 2002).

Since 1994, the Centers for Disease Control and Prevention (CDC) has attempted to define its mission in a more global context by taking a global approach to infectious diseases. CDC's strategy focuses on strengthening global capacity in six priority areas: international outbreak assistance, disease surveillance, applied research on diseases of global importance, application of proven public health tools, initiatives for disease control, and public health training for capacity building. This strategy can serve as a point of reference for the development of national, regional, and global strategies for addressing the globalization of infectious diseases.

Public–private partnerships serve as a vital conduit for providing public health care supplies and services to populations, particularly in the developing world, that would otherwise not receive them. Examples include a multitude of recently developed innovative, achievement-oriented joint venture collaborations and partnerships involving the privatization of health care delivery services, with the public sector setting the rules and monitoring the quality of service. These arrangements are characterized by their mutually beneficial nature and shared decision making, among other attributes. Yet despite the clear and growing demand for the participation of multinational corporations in these partnerships and in global health efforts in general, engaging their full interest still poses a considerable challenge. This situation is very worrisome. The Global Fund to Fight AIDS, Tuberculosis, and Malaria, for example, may not be sustainable without the commitment of nongovernmental entities, in terms of not only financing, but also technical and intellectual support.

Beyond a newer approach to infectious disease control on the part of the public health sector, globalization demands a new legal framework. The changing nature of the sovereignty and territorial basis of governments has tremendous implications for public health legislation and the role of international law in the prevention and control of emerging infectious diseases. International health regulations are being revised accordingly, but this may not be enough. Governance and the rule of law may have changed in such a way that even the revised regulations may not meet the legal needs of a new, internationally coordinated approach to the management of public health.

Finally, globalization demands a new social scientific framework for studying and understanding the emergence of infectious diseases. This is not a new realization. Five of the six factors related to the emergence of infectious diseases identified in a 1992 Institute of Medicine report on microbial threats (IOM, 1992) were social in nature, and the sixth, microbial adaptation and change, is partly the result of social behavior and social change. Yet the study of emerging infectious diseases is still conducted almost entirely within the realm of the biological sciences. The political ecology of disease might serve as new conceptual approach to studying and understanding the emergence of infectious diseases.

REFERENCES

CDC (Centers for Disease Control and Prevention). 2002. Tuberculosis morbidity among U.S.-born and foreign-born populations: United States, 2000. *MMWR* 51(05):101–104.

Cetron M. 2002 (April 16). *The World and Its Moving Parts*. Presentation at the Institute of Medicine Workshop on the Impact of Globalization on Infectious Disease Emergence and Control: Exploring the Consequences and Opportunities, Washington, D.C. Institute of Medicine Forum on Emerging Infections.

Corber S. 2002 (April 16). *Invited Discussion: A Response to the Shifting Trends*. Presentation at the Institute of Medicine Workshop on the Impact of Globalization on Infectious Disease Emergence and Control: Exploring the Consequences and Opportunities, Washington, D.C. Institute of Medicine Forum on Emerging Infections.

Echenberg M. 2002. *Black Death, White Medicine: Bubonic Plague and the Politics of Public Health in Colonial Senegal, 1914–1945*. Portsmouth, NH: Heinemann.

Friedman TL. 2000. *The Lexus and the Olive Tree: Understanding Globalization*. New York: Anchor Books.

Grondin D. 2002 (April 16). *Global Migration and Infectious Diseases*. Presentation at the Institute of Medicine Workshop on the Impact of Globalization on Infectious Disease Emergence and Control: Exploring the Consequences and the Opportunities, Washington, D.C. Institute of Medicine Forum on Emerging Infections.

IOM (Institute of Medicine). 1992. *Emerging Infections: Microbial Threats to Health in the United States*. Washington, D.C.: National Academy Press.

Klaucke D. 2002 (April 17). *Globalization and Health: A Framework for Analysis and Action.* Presentation at the Institute of Medicine Workshop on the Impact of Globalization on Infectious Disease Emergence and Control: Exploring the Consequences and the Opportunities, Washington, D.C. Institute of Medicine Forum on Emerging Infections.

Leaning J. 2002 (April 16). *Health, Human Rights, and Humanitarian Assistance: The Medical and Public Health Response to Crises and Disasters.* Presentation at the Institute of Medicine Workshop on The Impact of Globalization on Infectious Disease Emergence and Control: Exploring the Consequences and Opportunities, Washington, D.C. Institute of Medicine Forum on Emerging Infections.

Miller M. 2002 (April 17). *Invited Discussion: Considerations for Shaping the Agenda.* Presentation at the Institute of Medicine Workshop on the Impact of Globalization on Infectious Disease Emergence and Control: Exploring the Consequences and the Opportunities, Washington, D.C. Institute of Medicine Forum on Emerging Infections.

Mohle-Boetani JC, Werner SB, Waterman SH, Vugia DJ. 2000. The impact of health communication and enhanced laboratory-based surveillance on detection of cyclosporiasis outbreaks in California. *Emerging Infectious Diseases* 6(2):200–203.

Timpieri R. 2002 (April 17). *Invited Discussion: Considerations for Shaping the Agenda.* Presentation at the Institute of Medicine Workshop on the Impact of Globalization on Infectious Disease Emergence and Control: Exploring the Consequences and Opportunities, Washington, D.C. Institute of Medicine Forum on Emerging Infections.

WHO (World Health Organization). 1999. Infectious diseases are the biggest killer of the young. In: *Removing Obstacles to Healthy Development.* Geneva, Switzerland: WHO.

1

A World in Motion:
The Global Movement of People,
Products, Pathogens, and Power

Today, diseases as common as the cold and as rare as Ebola are circling the globe with near telephonic speed, making long-distance connections and intercontinental infections almost as if by satellite. You needn't even bother to reach out and touch someone. If you live, if you're homeothermic biomass, you will be reached and touched.

—Angier, 2001

The increasing cross-border and cross-continental movements of people, commodities, vectors, food, capital, and decision-making power that characterize globalization, together with global demographic trends, have enormous potential to affect the emergence and spread of infectious diseases. This chapter summarizes the workshop presentations and discussions on these various aspects of globalization and their implications for the prevention and control of emerging and reemerging infectious diseases.

The unprecedented volume and speed of human mobility are perhaps the most conspicuous manifestations of the present era of globalization. From international tourists to war-displaced refugees, more people are on the move than ever before. They are also traveling faster and are regularly visiting what used to be very remote parts of the world. This movement has the potential to change dramatically the factors involved in the transmission of infectious disease. Of particular concern, over the next 15 years, as the global population continues to grow and economic and social disparities between rich and poor countries intensify, the world will likely continue to witness rapidly growing numbers of migrants in search of employment or a better quality of life. In fact, many political scientists and demographers already refer to the twenty-first century as the "century of migration" (Leaning, 2002). Migrant populations are among the most vulnerable to emerging and reemerging infectious diseases and have been implicated as a key causal factor in the global spread of such diseases, most notably multidrug-resistant tuberculosis (TB). Workshop presentations and discussions addressing this increased human mobility and its effect on infectious disease transmission are summarized here; those addressing the need for improved surveillance of mobile populations are reported in Chapter 2.

Just as modern modes of transportation allow more people and products to travel around the world at a faster pace, they also open the airways to the transcontinental movement of infectious disease vectors. That mosquitoes can cross the ocean by riding in airplane wheel wells is a commonly cited example of this phenomenon and is one of several hypotheses proposed to explain the introduction of West Nile virus into New York City in 1999, the first known incidence of this disease in North America. Beyond such transport of disease vectors, controversial evidence suggests that global warming, much of which is generated by human activities, has caused or is causing changes in vector distributions worldwide and affecting the incidence rates of various tropical infectious diseases, such as malaria and dengue.

Consumers in much of the developed world expect constant access to a wide variety of high-quality, safe food products, regardless of the season or the product's geographic origin. This demand for a global food market and the resulting transnational movement of food have important implications for foodborne infectious diseases. The global transport of food also raises concerns about the risk of the emergence of antibiotic resistance in humans. Food-producing animals are often given antibiotic drugs for important therapeutic, disease prevention, or production reasons; however, these drugs can cause microbes to become resistant to drugs used to treat human illness.

Although the movement of people and products may be the most conspicuous manifestation of the present era of globalization, the phenomenon's main driving force is the global expansion of capitalism and the free-market system. Thus, it is useful to examine how the global flow of capital affects emerging and reemerging infectious diseases. The most direct effect results from the financing of environmental projects, such as dams and other water or land development efforts, that alter local vector ecologies and increase the potential for human exposure to infectious diseases. The movement of capital is often accompanied by movements or shifts in decision-making power, another manifestation of globalization with implications for infectious disease transmission.

The following sections address in turn each of these aspects of globalization and its implications for the transmission and spread of infectious disease. The last section summarizes the workshop presentation on the geographic spread of HIV/AIDS. As one participant argued, not only is the HIV/AIDS pandemic a devastating example of how global forces can cause or alter the emergence and spread of infectious disease, but, given its public health and economic impacts, it should probably also be a particular focus of any dialogue on global public health.

THE MOVEMENT OF PEOPLE[1]

A century and a half ago, it took about 365 days to circumnavigate the globe by ship; today it takes less than 36 hours. Thus the incubation period of many infectious diseases is now longer than the time it takes the infected to travel from one location to another. In the past, infectious disease outbreaks were readily detected on ships as they pulled into port, and the ships were quarantined until the diseases had burned themselves out. Now, should a local outbreak spread silently and globally via an infected traveler or tourist, cases will likely start emerging only days or weeks later in clinics and communities worldwide. Human movement has become a process that involves much more than what happens during the trip itself; the impact persists long afterward, particularly with regard to HIV, TB, and other latent infections.

In the meantime, the world's population has grown exponentially and more people have been on the move than ever before, especially during the past decade. According to Cetron (2002) migration volumes increased fourfold for the period 1960 through the 1990s. In 2001, an estimated 800 million people traveled; were forcibly displaced; or moved to new countries to work, study, join family members, or escape persecution. These individuals included international travelers (698 million), migrant workers (70–80 million), refugees and uprooted people (22 million), undocumented migrants (10–15 million), and migrant victims of human trafficking (0.7 million). This explosion in the rate of human mobility is almost certainly how HIV was introduced into North America and how fluoroquinolone-resistant gonococci were introduced into North America from Asia.

One participant noted that people on the move not only transmit infectious diseases, but also spread antimicrobial-resistant genetic material. A traveler's immunological system may afford protection from certain strains but not others. Thus, although there is a tendency to think of travelers as targets for infectious disease per se, it was suggested that perhaps they should also be thought of as interactive biological agents that pick up microbes and drug-resistant microbial genetic material in one part of the world and transport them to another. Although the global spread of drug-resistant microbes was not discussed at length during the workshop, with the exception of multidrug-resistant TB (an especially acute problem in Russia), the globalization of antimicrobial-resistant pathogens was identified as a serious, major issue. Another recent Forum workshop, Issues of

---

[1]This section is based on the workshop presentations by Cetron (2002), Grondin (2002), Mayer (2002), and Wilson (2002).

Resistance: Microbes, Vectors, and the Host, held in February 2002, was devoted to this topic.

International Travel

International travel is one of the fastest-growing industries worldwide; yearly international tourist arrivals are expected to pass the one billion mark by 2010. Every region of the world is experiencing this increase. An estimated 700 million tourists cross international borders each year. About 60 million people from other countries travel annually to the United States; around the same number of U.S. citizens travel internationally and then return. Between July 1998 and June 1999, the three New York City area airports experienced nearly five million international arrivals. The most rapid increases in international air travel, however, have been in Africa and the Middle East, places where many new infectious diseases are emerging.

Not only do international travelers themselves pose the risk of spreading infectious disease, but the airplanes on which they travel and the cargo that accompanies them also serve as potential sources of vector introduction. Decades ago, international arrivals were subject to vector spraying (i.e., inside the cabin, before the passengers exited the aircraft); participants suggested that it may not be long before routine vector surveillance on airplanes is reinstated. Beyond increasing the risk of the global spread of accidentally introduced infectious disease, international travel also increases society's vulnerability to acts of terrorism and their potentially devastating economic, psychological, and social repercussions. Part of the impact of the terrorist attacks on September 11, 2001, stemmed from the fact that air travel had until then been taken for granted. When a vehicle used for everyday business was turned into a weapon of destruction and terror, society was psychologically disrupted, and people's level of comfort with air travel has now declined.

Like air travel, cruise ship travel has increased dramatically, with nearly seven million people in North America traveling by this mode annually. In addition, although cruise ships are increasing in size and becoming more complex in design, they are still fairly densely populated. The average duration of stay on one of these ships is about two average incubation periods, which range from three to 10 days, for the microorganisms responsible for many emerging infectious diseases. These "floating cities," where people gather from all over the world for short periods of time, represent a unique environment for disease transmission, amplification, and dispersal (see Figure 1-1). Large aggregates of tourist populations not only serve as a potential source for the rapid spread of disease, but are also very difficult to monitor. Moreover, while the travelers on board a cruise ship are at risk of contracting infectious diseases, the people with whom they come into con-

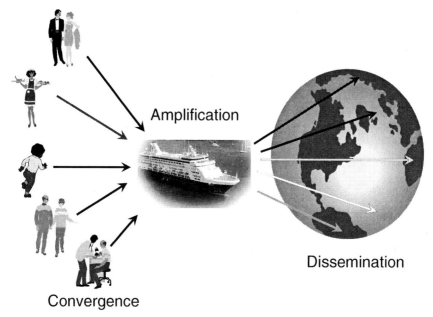

FIGURE 1-1   Cruise ship paradigm.
SOURCE: Cetron (2002).

tact when they leave the ship are also at risk. For example, the 1999 outbreak of influenza A virus Sydney in Alaska, which affected about 30,000 people, was preceded by the introduction of an influenza A virus Sydney strain via a cruise ship the previous year (IOM, 2005). It would therefore behoove all nations to be mindful of the ongoing threat of pandemic influenza and the fact that flu strains spread by cruise ships could be an important point of introduction.

Migration and Migrant Health

A 1998 *National Geographic* article describes human migration as "the dynamic undertow of population change; everyone's solution, everyone's conflict" (Parfit and Kasmauski, 1998, p. 11). Migration is propelled by a complex, dynamic interplay of various push and pull factors. Push factors are events such as war, strife, persecution, and famine that drive populations out of regions; pull factors are lures such as peace, freedom, sustenance, economic opportunity, and pleasure that cause populations to move to new locations. This section summarizes the workshop discussions on the latter factors; Chapter 2 summarizes the discussions on forced migration as a consequence of globally driven communal armed conflict.

The four major immigrant-receiving countries are the United States, Canada, Australia, and, more recently, Israel; European countries are seeing waves of immigration as well. The United States is experiencing the third-largest wave of immigration in history—twice as large as the previous peak, which occurred at the turn of the last century. Over the last 30 years, the number of foreign-born individuals in the United States has tripled. Over the past 10 years, 70 percent of U.S. population growth has been due to new Americans, including both direct immigrants (11.2 million people) and children born to immigrants (6.4 million). By 2000, 10.4 percent of the U.S. population (28.4 million) were foreign-born; of these, 51 percent were from Latin America, 25 percent from Asia, 15 percent from Europe, and the remainder from elsewhere.

In addition to individuals seeking permanent residency or citizenship status, migrant labor and work obtained through temporary work visas are significant sources of human movement, particularly between the United States and Mexico. There are an estimated 400 million legal northbound crossings annually along the 2,000-mile-long border between these two nations.

The United States is a nation of immigrants, a legacy that accounts for the country's economic prosperity and cultural diversity. Although that legacy must be recognized, the health of immigrants, their neighbors, and all populations in U.S. communities must be protected. Migrant health has emerged as a major, unresolved public health issue worldwide, especially in those countries that receive immigrants. Susceptibility to infection usually increases during transit and while living in the destination country, particularly if individuals are separated from their families, partners, or the social and cultural norms to which they are accustomed and that guide behavior in a stable community.

Recent trends in TB, particularly the incidence of multidrug-resistant TB, demonstrate the critical relationship between emerging infectious diseases and population mobility. TB has reemerged as the world's leading curable infectious killer. An estimated one-third of the world's population is infected with *Mycobacterium tuberculosis*, the organism that causes the disease. A three percent increase in new TB cases occurs every year, and approximately 10 percent of these infections develop into active disease. If left untreated, a single infectious person can infect as many as 10 to 15 other people each year.

Fully 95 percent of TB cases occur in the developing world, with a 10 percent increase in Africa being due to coinfection with HIV. (People coinfected with HIV and TB are up to 800 times more likely to develop active TB, and TB kills 15 percent of HIV-infected persons.) TB is reemerging even in the developed world, however, where its prevalence has previously been low, largely because of migration from poorer, high-prevalence countries. In Russia, for example, TB has become the leading cause of death from infectious and parasitic diseases; although the reasons are unclear, immigration is probably an important factor.

Countries that receive migrants generally report that although the number of TB cases among their domestically born populations has declined or stabilized over the last 10 years, the number of cases among their foreign-born populations has increased.

- In the United States, more than 50 percent of new TB cases occur in foreign-born populations. Between 1995 and 1998, the decrease in TB case rates among people born in the United States was three and a half times that of people born elsewhere.
- A 1994 British study showed that the incidence of reported active TB in entrant populations was 20 times higher than the national incidence (Rieder et al., 1994).
- In Denmark, the number of cases of TB has doubled in the past decade, mostly because of immigration (Dragsted et al., 1999).
- In Australia, the prevalence of TB among immigrants is comparable to that in each immigrant's home country and much higher than that in Australia.
- On the basis of preliminary data from a 2000 International Organization for Migration health assessment of more than 76,000 migrants and refugees, the TB incidence rate among migrant populations is generally five to six times higher than the average rates among the populations of the countries of destination (i.e., the United States, Canada, and Australia); these findings are consistent with reports from the host countries.

Receiving countries of migrants also report increased occurrence of multidrug-resistant TB in their foreign-born populations. Up to 92 percent of such cases in Canada, 90 percent of such cases in Australia, and 76 percent of such cases in the Netherlands were among foreign-born individuals.

The majority (61 percent) of migrants with active TB requiring treatment come from Southeast Asia, corresponding to an incidence of 1,235 per 100,000 population; this figure is eight to nine times higher than the reported cumulative prevalence rates of these countries based on 1999 World Health Organization data. According to other recent estimates, countries with the highest number of annual new multidrug-resistant TB cases worldwide include India (238,806), China (158,813), Russia (11,430), Peru (2,906), Ivory Coast (2,190), Argentina (1,598), Brazil (1,591), Zimbabwe (1,508), South Korea (1,233), Romania (985), Dominican Republic (794), and Sierra Leone (586).

Several factors account for the extreme vulnerability of mobile populations to infectious disease: lack of access to health care and social services in the receiving countries; the conditions and structures of the migration process itself, including social instability, poverty, powerlessness, discrimination, sexual exploitation, and the absence or paucity of social and legal protections; and behavioral changes that are typical of mobile populations. The problem is compounded by the polarity that exists within the health care community: on the one hand, efforts are being made to cure illnesses for which migrant patients are seeking care, but on the other hand, the same health care providers are being asked to screen individuals who are at tremendous risk if the outcome of the screening process is unfavorable. Most migrants generally have no desire to be screened or to visit a health care provider, even when they are experiencing problems, and they often avoid making or keeping appointments as a result. Gaining their trust and convincing them that health care and screening are to their benefit is difficult but necessary. If, for example, individuals do not tell their providers that they are being treated for TB—or worse, if they have stopped treatment—they may not receive adequate, continued care. In addition, many undocumented migrants will not seek medical care because of their illegal status and the risk of being reported to immigration authorities, or even deported.

The United States and other developed nations are not in an ideal position to receive the massive influx of migrants. This is true not only from a public health perspective (e.g., see Chapter 2 for a discussion of mobile health screening and surveillance efforts), but also because of growing tensions between residents and "foreigners" that are creating an in-group versus out-group social phenomenon. Even though individual countries have made liberal and humane attempts to adapt to the influx of people, political and human interactions are becoming more difficult because of this growing tension, particularly in Europe.

GLOBAL DEMOGRAPHIC TRENDS[2]

Changing world demographics, especially the rapidly increasing size of the world's population, play a key role in the impact of globalization on the emergence and spread of infectious diseases. In fact, as one participant emphasized, the dynamic interplay between poverty and global population growth is the single most important factor responsible for many infectious disease problems. Even though global population growth is declining at an

---

[2]This section is based on the workshop presentations by Cetron (2002), Cleghorn (2002), Corber (2002), Gordon (2002), Leaning (2002), LeDuc (2002), Widdus (2002), and Wilson (2002).

ever-increasing rate, there will still be a billion more people living on the planet by 2015. As detailed in *Global Trends 2015* (NIC, 2001), other important global demographic trends that will likely have a direct impact on infectious disease threats include increasing urbanization in poor countries, the growth of the developed world's aging population (see below), the demographic consequences of the HIV/AIDS pandemic, and the growing proportion of youth in poor countries. All of these trends are expected to have profound effects on the already sharp demographic and public health disparities between rich and poor countries and fuel even more migration, both legal and illegal, from poor to rich countries.

Diverging Age Distributions

Fully 95 percent of the population growth that is expected to occur over the next 15 years will be in poor countries, especially in urban areas. Meanwhile, population growth rates in rich countries are declining rapidly, and as noted, the proportion of elderly populations in these countries is increasing significantly. This is especially true in Europe and Japan, as elaborated at the April 2002 United Nations Conference on Aging, but it is also the case in the United States. As a result, it is expected that spending on health care for the elderly will threaten to crowd out spending in other areas; there will be intense political pressure from aging cohorts to fund research on treatments for diseases associated with aging rather than on the prevention and control of infectious diseases associated with youth. Garnering the willingness and capability to devote the necessary resources to infectious diseases, particularly those that affect poor regions of the world, will be a political challenge.

The major causes of death in the poorest 20 percent of the world's population are AIDS, respiratory diseases, diarrheal diseases, and a range of other infectious diseases. In fact, infectious diseases, many of which are associated with youth, are responsible for 80 percent of the differences in the causes of death between the poorest 20 percent and the richest 20 percent of the world's population—in other words, the excess premature deaths that occur in the poorest parts of the world. An increasing proportion of youth in poor countries is another major global demographic feature expected to emerge by 2015, stemming in part from the profound impact of the global AIDS epidemic on the age distribution of the populations in the hardest-hit countries.

Urbanization in Poor Countries

Urbanization in poor countries is expected to become a key demographic feature of the world over the next 15 years, as more than 90 percent of the population growth in poor countries will be in cities. Already, about half of the world's population lives in urban areas—more than ever before. By contrast, in most parts of the developed world (e.g., in the eastern United States), the size of the urban population is not expected to change substantially over the next 30 years.

The increasing urbanization in poor countries has significant implications for the transmission and spread of infectious disease.

• About two-thirds of all fatal infectious diseases are spread person to person; greater population density increases transmission by bringing people into closer contact with each other.

• The stress on already weak health systems in many poor countries is increasing.

• Water and sanitation systems are weak or lacking in many urban areas of poor countries, thus increasing susceptibility to contaminated waterborne diseases.

• The huge periurban slums that tend to develop around many major cities in developing countries are typically poor areas that lack infrastructure and resources. This, combined with the warm weather and low latitudes of most of these regions, makes these slums ideal sites for the spread of infectious diseases.

• Because urban centers serve as stopping-off points for international travelers, an infectious traveler could potentially and unknowingly set off a worldwide epidemic. More than 5,000 urban center airports worldwide have regularly scheduled international flights.

• Urban areas in poor countries also serve as temporary or permanent residences for the many people who migrate from their rural homes in search of work; an infected migrant could spread a disease that might otherwise have been locally contained.

The worldwide resurgence of dengue illustrates the impact urban growth can have on the emergence of infectious disease. Sustained transmission of the dengue virus requires a population of between about 150,000 and one million people. A growing number of subtropical and tropical urbanized areas are becoming large enough to favor the ongoing transmission of one or more of the four dengue serotypes. These areas are typically littered with many discarded, nonbiodegradable items (e.g., glass, plastic, and old tires) that provide ideal vector breeding sites. In fact, *Aedes aegypti*, which carries both the dengue and yellow fever viruses, lives almost exclusively in cohabitation with humans; one could even say that humans have evolved to serve this mosquito since they so readily provide it with the means to propagate. Urbanization, combined with the subtropical and tropical temperatures that favor viral mobility (the extrinsic incubation period is

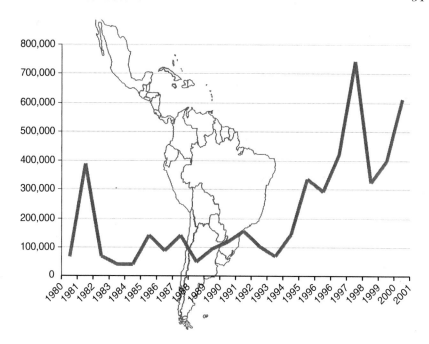

FIGURE 1-2   Dengue cases, 1980–2001.
SOURCE: Corber (2002).

shorter in warmer areas), creates a perfect setting for the emergence of
dengue.

Dengue has caused massive epidemics in the United States in the past;
however, it has not reemerged because current living conditions, including
the use of screens and air conditioning, limit its transmission. Interestingly,
in 1985 another vector, *Aedes albopictus*, was introduced into the United
States, and since then it has spread to at least 12 states via used tires.
Dengue has, moreover, reemerged with a vengeance in most of the rest of
the Americas, where the number of cases has risen from only a few to nearly
one million (see Figure 1-2). Not surprisingly, its reemergence coincides
with the environmental presence of glass, plastics, and tires. This region is
witnessing all four dengue serotypes, all of which can cause illness and have
caused pandemics in the past. When individuals are infected with any of the
serotypes for the first time, they usually develop classic dengue, a less severe
form of the disease. Once they have been infected with another serotype,
however, they are at risk for a more severe form of the disease; infection
with one serotype offers no protection against another. One of the more
severe forms of the disease, dengue hemorrhagic fever, or dengue shock

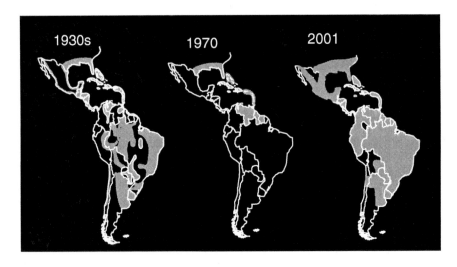

FIGURE 1-3   Reinfestation of *Aedes aegypti.*
SOURCE: Corber (2002).

syndrome, is one of the worst possible outcomes and has about a 10 percent mortality rate. The Caribbean is experiencing an epidemic of DEN-3, a dengue virus serotype that has not been present in the area for the past 30 years and that was recently reintroduced from Asia. Because the Caribbean has experienced epidemics involving other serotypes, the likelihood that dengue hemorrhagic fever will appear in the region over the next few years is even greater than it would otherwise be.

Although infection with dengue virus is not associated with HIV/AIDS, as far as is known, it does cause activation of certain cell surface molecules (HLA class II molecules). This phenomenon may play a role in the HIV/AIDS epidemic in the Caribbean by providing HIV with more cellular targets to attack. This may explain why the average time interval between HIV infection and the onset of AIDS is shorter in the Caribbean, where the recent emergence of dengue is a major public health problem, than in North America and Europe (Cleghorn, 2002).

The history of dengue in the Caribbean demonstrates how a false sense of security can breed reemergence. In the 1930s it was believed that if *Aedes aegypti* could be eradicated, so, too, could disease. Although a number of countries participated in eradication efforts and had achieved local success by about 1970, not all countries participated, and the mosquito was not entirely eradicated from the region (see Figure 1-3). However, because the numbers of mosquitoes had diminished in most areas and because funding had dried up, surveillance ceased. As a result, over the last 30 years, with

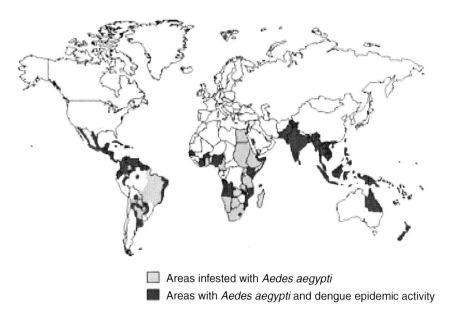

☐ Areas infested with *Aedes aegypti*
■ Areas with *Aedes aegypti* and dengue epidemic activity

FIGURE 1-4 World distribution of dengue, 2005.
SOURCE: CDC (2005).

the increasing intensity of globalizing forces such as trade and travel, *Aedes aegypti* has reinfested nearly every country in the American region except for Canada (see Figure 1-4).

THE MOVEMENT OF VECTORS[3]

Increased vector movement may be just as important as increased human movement in contributing to the global spread of infectious diseases. There is perhaps no better illustration of this point than the global spread of *Aedes aegypti* and the worldwide resurgence of dengue, as described above. This same mosquito has also been responsible for yellow fever outbreaks worldwide; endemic zones include every country in South America except for Brazil (see Figure 1-5a) and more than half the countries in Africa (see Figure 1-5b).

---

[3]This section is based on the workshop presentations by Cetron (2002) and Mayer (2002).

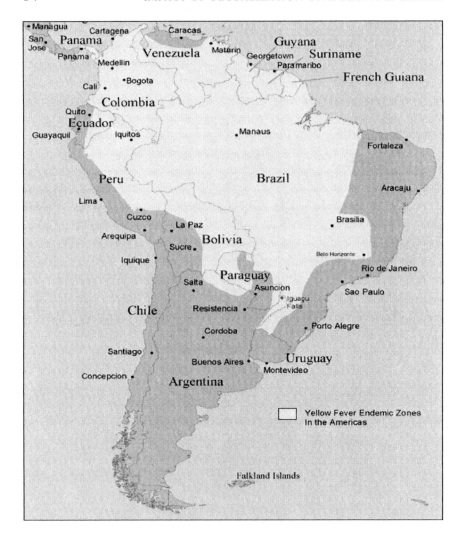

FIGURE 1-5a   Yellow fever-endemic zones in the Americas, 2005.
SOURCE: CDC (2005).

Vectors are usually introduced into new areas inadvertently via vehicles used to transport people or commodities (e.g., airplanes) or via commodities that are being transported. It has been demonstrated experimentally that a number of different disease vectors can survive in the wheel wells of jet aircraft at high altitudes for long intercontinental flights. Mosquitoes also hitchhike on used car tires that are being transported for retreading or other purposes. For example, the Asian tiger mosquito, *Aedes albopictus*, a dengue

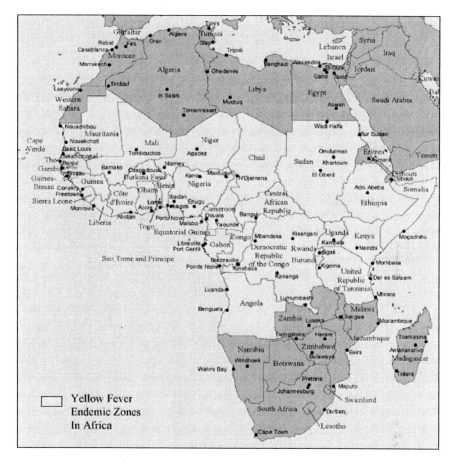

FIGURE 1-5b   Yellow fever-endemic zones in Africa, 2005.
SOURCE: CDC (2005).

virus vector, was introduced to the North American continent on rubber tires shipped to Houston. The United States–Mexico border, a dumping ground for used tires, is an important breeding site for *Aedes* mosquitoes.

Animal importations are another potential source of introduced zoonoses. Each year many U.S. ports of entry receive millions of animal importations from countries where a variety of diseases are endemic. In a single year (i.e., August 1998 to July 1999), there were more than 2.8 million international animal importations into New York City; most of these were amphibians (61 percent) and birds (36 percent). In 1996, the port of Miami received more than 30 million animal imports, most of which (96 percent) were fish and aquatic invertebrates. It should be noted, moreover, that these figures represent only legally imported animals and that a large trade in illegally imported animals exists as well.

Before its first appearance in New York City in 1999, West Nile virus was not present in the western hemisphere. It has now spread throughout the North American continent, into Canada, Mexico, Central America, and the Caribbean. This example of the potential for the introduction of a vectorborne infectious disease into a new hemisphere also illustrates how a multitude of factors can converge to provide a ripe opportunity for emergence: the most common vector of West Nile virus in the United States, the common household mosquito (*Culex pipiens*), was already ubiquitous in the New York metropolitan area; the marshy habitat where the disease emerged was an ideal mosquito breeding ground; the location of emergence was near a major international airport; and international travelers are constantly arriving in Queens, which houses perhaps one of the most ethnically diverse populations in the world.

Although the virus was almost certainly introduced via a transportation vehicle, it is unclear whether it was introduced via a vector mosquito or some other means. Other possibilities include the arrival of an infected human, an infected bird on an airplane or other transportation vehicle, an infected migrating bird, or an infected animal reservoir in the New York City area. At this point, there may be no way to trace the precise means of introduction, which in any case is somewhat immaterial, as the virus is well established in animal populations and has spread rapidly down the East Coast of the United States.

Effects of Global Temperature Change on Vector Movement

Few would argue at this point in time that global warming is occurring and is generated primarily by human activities. Conclusive evidence suggests that industrialization, the burning of fossil fuels for heat and transportation, and deforestation cause global warming by increasing the levels of greenhouse gasses and eliminating carbon sinks. It is also known that many aspects of vector behavior, including the range of habitability, are at least partially driven by temperature. Thus, there is some concern that as global temperatures rise, vectorborne diseases could spread to areas where they have not previously existed (i.e., they would move north in the northern hemisphere, south in the southern hemisphere, and higher in mountainous areas).

However, empirical studies investigating changes in the distribution of vectors and vectorborne diseases due to global warming have yielded highly contradictory results. Some studies have shown that higher temperatures have led to increased rates of malaria, dengue, and other vectorborne diseases in temperate areas; others have not. Moreover, although temperature-dependent mathematical models predict that the prevalence of vectors and vectorborne diseases, particularly malaria, will increase in temperate zones and at higher altitudes as temperatures rise, multivariate models incorporating other variables, such as rainfall and humidity, show that higher temperatures do not necessarily result in increased incidence and global redistribution of mosquito vectors (Rogers and Randolph, 2000). In fact, the worldwide incidence of malaria may actually decrease with global warming, as many climatic factors that accompany higher temperatures appear to counteract the effects of temperature; for example, the increased rainfall that often accompanies higher temperatures could wash out the breeding pools of anopheline mosquitoes. Some scientists who believe that the resurgence of malaria in the East African highlands is not climate related argue that the resurgence is more likely associated with other factors, such as declining surveillance and treatment (Hay et al., 2002).

El Niño Southern Oscillations (ENSOs) would appear to provide a natural opportunity for investigating the effects of increased temperature and rainfall fluctuations on the incidence of vectorborne diseases. Because the phenomenon lasts only one to two years, however, it is difficult to extrapolate ENSO findings to global warming. The social, architectural, and engineering adaptations that would be expected to occur with increased global warming cannot take place during such short time periods. Over the next century, when temperatures worldwide are expected to increase by as much as 5–10°C, human behavior will likely change in unforeseen ways. Moreover, as with other studies of the effects of temperature changes, the results of studies of ENSO-related temperature increases are contradictory: some studies suggest that temperature increases do in fact lead to greater incidence of malaria, dengue, and other diseases in Africa, Asia, and elsewhere, but others show that there is very little change.

As important as it is to take a global perspective, it is also very difficult to make global generalizations about diseases, such as malaria, that are so shaped by local conditions and could emerge under any of an infinite variety of local circumstances. As Hackett (1937, p. 226) observed: "Everything about malaria is so molded by local conditions that it becomes a thousand epidemiological puzzles. Like chess, it is played with a few pieces but is capable of an infinite variety of situations." Malaria is transmitted by dozens of anopheline species; some breed preferentially in warmer temperatures, whereas others prefer cooler temperatures and cannot even survive in warmer conditions. Mathematical–spatial models generally lack sufficient geographic resolution to account for local ecological conditions.

The Movement of Livestock

Although the movement of livestock is not recognized as a cause of zoonotic diseases, it was cited by workshop participants as an important manifestation of globalization with significant economic and psychological impacts. The emergence of foot-and-mouth disease in England wiped out an entire market, closed export doors, and had devastating economic consequences. It also had a tremendous psychological impact; indeed, it resulted in a number of suicides. In one case, a third-generation cattle breeder had just received an award in the mail for having the number-one herd in England; his cattle were killed later that day. The outbreak also affected health care, schooling, and food distribution in general. If foot-and-mouth disease were introduced into the United States, either accidentally or intentionally, the consequences would be devastating, both economically and psychologically.

Direct contact with livestock and other animals can also have an impact on human health. Between September 1998 and June 1999, a large outbreak of encephalitis occurred among pig farmers in Malaysia, and Nipah virus was identified as the causal agent. There were 265 cases of the illness reported to the Malaysian Ministry of Health, including more than 100 deaths. Transmission of the Nipah virus to humans occurs primarily through direct contact with infected pigs or swine tissue; no evidence of human-to-human transmission has been found. As a result of this outbreak, more than 900,000 pigs were culled.

Livestock are used and moved around for other reasons besides food. Too often people forget how closely they are interrelated with animals through the use of animal products, from leather shoes to cosmetics. The United States was very concerned, for example, about the importation of gluten by-products, which are included in cosmetics and other products, during the European outbreak of bovine spongiform encephalophy (mad cow disease) in the 1990s.

THE MOVEMENT OF FOOD[4]

The way people eat is changing the way food is transported around the world. In the 1950s, supermarket shelves were filled with hundreds of items; today they are filled with tens of thousands of food products from all over the world. Consumers expect to be able to choose from a wide range of safe, high-quality food items, including fresh meat and produce, year-round. To meet these expectations, the food industry must import items from many different parts of the world. A globalized food supply raises questions about food safety and opens the door for potential bioterrorist attacks. For example, are people being exposed to new and different pathogens? What factors can lead to an increased risk of infectious disease under

---

[4]This section is based on the workshop presentations by Acheson (2002) and Kimball (2002).

these circumstances? What controls are in place to manage this potential risk? The globalization of the food supply also raises many important questions about antibiotic resistance. For instance, what drugs are being used to treat food animals? What local controls exist? What effect does the indiscriminate use of antibiotics in certain parts of the world have on enteric pathogens that may enter the United States (or other countries) through the food supply?

Several hundred known foodborne microbial agents, including bacteria, viruses, and parasites, pose potential dangers everywhere in the world, including the United States. Added to these are a multitude of chemical hazards (i.e., antibiotics, carcinogens, and heavy metals), physical hazards, prions, allergens, and various other agents that threaten human health. New food-transmitted agents are continually being identified. Threats identified since 1977 include *Campylobacter jejuni*; *Campylobacter fetus subsp. fetus*; *Cryptosporidium parvum*; *Cyclospora cayetanensis*; Shiga toxin-producing *Escherichia coli*; *Listeria monocytogenes*; noroviruses[5]; *Salmonella bongori*; *Salmonella enterica* serovar *Enteritidis*; *Salmonella enterica* serovar *Typhimurium*; transmissible spongiform encephalopathic agents; *Vibrio cholerae* O139; *Vibrio vulnificus*; *Vibrio parahaemolyticus*; and *Yersinia enterocolitica*. Although all of these potential hazards occur worldwide, some, such as parasites, are more problematic in some areas than in others. No one country or community has the capability to test for all possible hazardous agents in its imported food products, which makes local control very important.

Each year, a growing number of different foods are imported into countries throughout the world. Recent outbreaks have demonstrated the impact of imported produce on the occurrence of foodborne disease. In 1998, for example, an outbreak of multidrug-resistant *Shigella sonnei* infection occurred among patrons of restaurants in Minnesota (CDC, 1999). The culprit in this case was imported parsley.

Guatemalan raspberries are a classic example of a cash crop that is introduced into a poor country with unsafe cultivation practices and then reintroduced into the North American market as a contaminated fresh produce item. A herald wave of 35 cases of cyclosporiasis occurred in 1996, followed by about 1,400 cases the next year, with clusters occurring in both the United States and Canada. Careful case-controlled studies determined that the outbreaks were associated with contaminated raspberries; laboratory-confirmed cases demonstrated that the clusters occurred seasonally, following the importation of Guatemalan raspberries. At the end of May 1997, the Guatemalan Berry Commission voluntarily

---

[5]Formerly known as Norwalk-like viruses.

suspended shipments of raspberries to the North American market, and the impact was profound: the outbreaks ceased. The following year, however, even though the commission had imposed voluntary controls on cultivation (because it was believed that contaminated groundwater had been used to spread insecticides on the raspberry plants, and there was no way to decontaminate the berries), Canada continued to import the raspberries and continued to experience cyclosporiasis outbreaks. The United States, on the other hand, prohibited the importation of Guatemalan raspberries and experienced no further outbreaks. As this example demonstrates, local conditions, local controls, and import controls all play significant roles in the prevention and control of outbreaks of foodborne disease.

Local conditions set the stage for a pathogen to enter the food supply. The health of the workforce, the health of animals, local sanitary conditions, process controls in the food production plant, water quality, and refrigeration control all play a role. Of these, workforce health and local sanitary conditions are the most critical; both are believed to have contributed to the 1996–1998 cyclosporiasis outbreak. The presence of parasites in either the water or the workforce has also been implicated in cryptosporidiosis and giardiasis outbreaks, while bacterial agents in either the water or the workforce have been associated with diseases caused by vibrios and other enteric organisms.

From the perspective of the U.S Department of Agriculture, local inspectors are responsible for safeguarding their food exports. In 1999 and 2000, there were 5,972 inspectors in the 34 countries exporting food products to the United States, including 1,493 inspectors in Canada, 504 in Australia, 586 in Denmark, and 910 in New Zealand. The United States typically imports 2.4–2.8 billion pounds of meat and poultry annually. In fiscal year 2001, the United States imported food products from 33 different countries, with the amounts imported varying greatly by country. For example, more than 1,500 million pounds of meat and poultry was imported from Canada, but only 18,000 pounds from Switzerland. On the basis of 1999 data, most imports come from Canada (49 percent), Australia (22 percent), New Zealand (14 percent), and Denmark (four percent). Of these imports, 85 percent are fresh meat, 13 percent processed meat, and two percent poultry. The imports come from 1,200 authorized plants distributed among the 33 countries; more than 70 percent of these plants are in Canada (470), Italy (115), Denmark (100), Australia (99), and New Zealand (81).

A country wishing to export meat, poultry, or eggs to the United States must establish and maintain a two-step inspection system equivalent to that of the United States. First, the system must be assessed by means of a document review, which involves the evaluation of five risk factors: sanitation controls, animal disease controls, slaughter and processing controls, residue controls, and enforcement controls. If this first step is successful, the second is an onsite audit of the risk factors, plant facilities, equipment, laboratories, training programs, and in-plant inspection operations. Countries must be recertified annually, and the U.S. Food Safety and Inspection Service (FSIS) regularly conducts onsite audits to ensure that this system equivalency is maintained. Problems may lead to the suspension of eligibility.

All imported products require a foreign inspection certificate. When products arrive in the United States for importation, the following must be documented on the certificate: product name, establishment number, country of origin, name and address of manufacturer, quantity and weight of contents, list of ingredients, species of animal, and identification marks. Should a recall be necessary, this information allows control of the contaminated product. In addition, importers must file an entry form with the U.S. Customs Service within five days of product arrival.

FSIS also requires an original certificate from the country of origin indicating that the product has passed local inspection. Even after passing local inspection, all meat and poultry shipments must be held and reinspected upon arrival. This includes a visual inspection, certification check, and product examination for chemical or microbiological contamination. Egg products are reinspected at the processing facility, not at the holding warehouse.

Microorganisms for which tests are routinely conducted include *Listeria monocytogenes* and *Salmonella* in ready-to-eat foods; *Escherichia coli* O157:H7, *Salmonella*, *L. monocytogenes*, and *Staphylococcus aureus* in dried and semidried sausage; and *E. coli* O157:H7 in raw ground beef. Residue sampling plants randomly sample animal products for drug residues as part of the National Residue Program.

THE MOVEMENT OF CAPITAL[6]

The movement of capital refers, in its simplest sense, to the transferability of money and the increasing linkages within the world's financial system. While having received scant attention in the public health literature, the global flow of capital and the international unification of markets have been emphasized by social scientists and in the more economically oriented globalization literature. Their importance is reflected in the fact that the "development of global financial markets" is Soros's (2002) operational definition of globalization.

---

[6]This section is based on the workshop presentations by Mayer (2002) and Patz (2002).

In fact, many would argue that the movement of capital is a crucial component of the very definition of globalization. Although the term is commonly used to describe contemporary society, it is often ill defined and misunderstood (Buse and Walt, 2002). In the health sciences literature, it usually refers to the process of growing global interdependence, particularly as manifested by increasing international transportation; at least for social scientists, however, this interdependency is only part of the process of globalization. A workshop participant suggested that the health sciences field could benefit from an explicit understanding of the concept of globalization as developed in the literature in such fields as international relations, political economy, and political geography. As was noted in a recent article on the implications of the globalization of cholera for global governance, "This is a rich and highly relevant literature. It documents what structural changes are occurring toward a global political economy, how power relationships are embedded within this process of change, what varying impacts this may have on individuals and groups, and to what extent global governance could effectively mediate this process" (Lee and Dodson, 2000, p. 213). Globalization encompasses much more than an increase in international interdependency and connectivity; in particular, it also includes the movement of capital.

The most direct consequence of the international movement of capital for emerging infectious diseases is the financing of environmental projects in a country with external funds. These projects, frequently planned by a coalition of local and international environmental planners, usually have either intended or unintended environmental effects and alter human–environment relations in ways that have significant implications for host–pathogen interactions and potential human exposure to vectorborne or waterborne diseases.

Water Projects

Water projects perhaps provide the best example of how the global movement of capital affects the emergence and transmission of infectious disease as a result of the alteration of local conditions. The explicit purpose of dams and other water projects is to fuel local and regional economies through the generation of hydroelectric power, to generate new capital, and to integrate countries into the global economy. The massive Three Gorges Dam project, for example, is designed explicitly to power Chinese industrial growth and further China's position in the global economy. The costly construction of dams usually entails large investments of outside capital. Even when financing comes almost exclusively from domestic sources, as in the case of the Three Gorges Dam, at least some funding usually derives indirectly from business growth due to globalization.

The construction of dams has many known deleterious public health consequences. For example, construction of the Aswan Dam in Egypt has been implicated in increased rates of schistosomiasis (Abdel-Wahab, 1982; El Alamy and Cline, 1997). Likewise, the development of dams in the Senegal River basin is among the major factors leading to a significantly increased prevalence of schistosomiasis over a period of only three years (Gryseels et al., 1994). As another example, the construction and anticipated completion of the Three Gorges Dam—presumably the largest dam in the world and, some would suggest, the largest public works project in the history of the world—will almost certainly lead to the introduction of schistosomiasis. This concerns many scientists because schistosomiasis will be introduced into an area upstream of the dam where the disease is not endemic, where ecological conditions will be highly conducive to its transmission, and where human exposure is expected to be substantial. Moreover, construction of the Three Gorges Dam is resulting in massive population displacement, forced migration, and very high population densities in certain regions, all of which further increase the likelihood of the emergence of infectious disease.

Land Modification Projects

Land modification and clearance projects that involve capital flow can also have significant consequences for the emergence and transmission of infectious diseases through their alteration of local human–environment relations. For example, the clearance of land in Malaysia for the construction of rubber plantations, economic development, and the promotion of an export economy have resulted in notable increases in the rates of malaria transmission among plantation laborers. Environmental conditions have been altered to such an extent that the landscape has became conducive to anopheline mosquito breeding, and the level of human contact with anopheline mosquitoes has greatly increased.

As another example, deforestation in the Amazon, both for logging and for gold mining, has been linked to increased incidence of *Anopheles darlingi* mosquitoes, the primary vector of malaria in South America. These mosquitoes were not present in the area before the mid-1960s. The situation is exacerbated by the fact that mercury, which is used to extract gold from the ore, acts as an immunosuppressive agent, increasing the likelihood of contracting malaria (Patz, 2002; Silva et al., 2004). Moreover, the migration of laborers into and out of these areas contributes to the spread of disease throughout South America.

It should be noted that, although the clearing of land results in an increase in malaria in most instances, it can also lead to a decrease in the rate of malarial transmission. For example, the clearing of land in Thailand for tapioca farming led to a decrease in malarial transmission by destroying the habitat of the vector, *Anopheles dirus* (Bockarie and Paru, 1993).

THE MOVEMENT OF DECISION-MAKING POWER[7]

Workshop participants identified as another important manifestation of globalization shifts in the locus of power in global decision making, whereby some localities are marginalized in their ability to control what happens to local society and others have more central control and are able to project power over great distances. The increasing uniformity of society, the erosion of locally controlled commodities and markets, and the general loss of societal control all reflect these shifts in power.

It is this dimension of globalization—the shift in decision-making power—that is so politically controversial and was responsible for protests at the World Trade Organization's meeting in Seattle in 1999 (Sassen, 1998). Although many people, such as Friedman (2000), perceive globalization as a phenomenon that promotes well-being and economic opportunity, others view it as an alienating social force that marginalizes those already at the periphery of society. Even if one does not agree with the latter sentiment, a workshop participant suggested that it might be helpful to understand this perspective, as it may elucidate the nature of some of the underlying social factors in the global emergence of infectious diseases. Ultimately, these underlying social factors—including poverty, population growth, and the massive displacement of people—must be addressed to ensure a sustainable global capacity to prevent and control the emergence and spread of infectious diseases.

THE GEOGRAPHIC EVOLUTION OF HIV/AIDS[8]

Not only does the global spread of HIV/AIDS serve as a paradigm for the effect of globalization on emerging infectious diseases, but HIV/AIDS has also emerged as an overriding concern because it makes people more susceptible to other infectious diseases, particularly TB. Because of its economic impact, moreover, it has a major effect on the absorptive capacities of the public health systems of developing countries. In fact, as one workshop participant noted, most global health issues can truly be understood only within the larger context of the HIV/AIDS pandemic.

Since its emergence in the early-1980s, HIV has infected about 60

---

[7]This section is based on the workshop presentation by Mayer (2002).
[8]This section is based on the workshop presentation by Gordon (2002).

million people worldwide, 40 million of whom were estimated still to be living by the end of 2001. The global spread of HIV is attributed mainly to the movement of people.

Even though southern Africa and the Great Lakes region of eastern Africa remain the areas of the world hardest hit by the HIV/AIDS pandemic, growing rates of infection in other areas, particularly elsewhere in Africa, are of increasing concern. Nigeria and Ethiopia, the largest African countries, may be at a point where the epidemic is about to become much more serious over the next five years. If this is the case and if the situation in Nigeria and Ethiopia parallels that of southern Africa in the early 1990s, it is not inconceivable that the number of HIV/AIDS cases in Africa could double in the next five years.

The current official HIV/AIDS rate in Nigeria is six percent, but it is likely that the real number is closer to 10 percent. The Nigerian government has shown some commitment to dealing with the problem, but there has been very little progress in terms of destigmatization. Continuing social, political, and economic tensions associated with this highly populated nation are diverting attention away from the threat of AIDS.

In other parts of the world, India has the greatest potential for a widespread increase in the number of people with HIV/AIDS, given that 70 to 80 percent of the population lives in poor rural areas where the education rates are low and the public health infrastructure is weak. HIV/AIDS is already costing India substantially in terms of lost productivity and treatment costs.

Although Russia has one of the fastest-growing rates of HIV infection in the world, with the number of official cases roughly doubling each year since 1998, it is not facing quite the same level of threat as the countries of sub-Saharan Africa and India. The rapid spread of HIV into Russia, as well as Ukraine, has been associated with the opening up of the Eastern European countries and the subsequent movement of people between zones where the populations have various rates of HIV infection. Most new infections in Russia appear to be linked to injection drug use, but several other factors—including high rates of unemployment, a disintegrating public health infrastructure, and the general poor status of health care services—make the country vulnerable to further increases. On the other hand, given the high rate of literacy and general education throughout Russia, there is reason for optimism. Russia's extensive media links could be used to develop an active education program that could have a significant impact in a fairly short period of time. The country's demographic profile, which is skewed toward an older population, is also likely to blunt the impact of HIV/AIDS.

The Chinese government and news media have recently focused much more attention on HIV/AIDS than in the past, suggesting that the situation is worrisome and that the government is becoming aware of the potential risks. Still, China has far to go in terms of acknowledging the scope of the problem. Officially, 850,000 people in China are infected with HIV, but this number is obviously far at odds with reality.

The spread of HIV/AIDS, both in sub-Saharan Africa and elsewhere, is likely to hinder prospects for a transition to democracy by undermining civil society, hampering the evolution of sound political and economic institutions, and polarizing the struggle for power and the control of resources in poor countries.

REFERENCES

Abdel-Wahab MF. 1982. *Schistosomiasis in Egypt*. Boca Raton, FL: CRC Press, Inc.

Acheson D. 2002 (April 16). *Globalization of the Food Supply*. Presentation at the Institute of Medicine Workshop on the Impact of Globalization on Infectious Disease Emergence and Control: Exploring the Consequences and Opportunities, Washington, D.C. Institute of Medicine Forum on Emerging Infections.

Angier N. 2001, May 6. Together, in Sickness and in Health. *New York Times Magazine*. http://www.nytimes.com/2001/05/06/magazine/06INTRO.html [accessed on January 18, 2006].

Bockarie MJ, Paru R. 1993. *Forest Clearing, Mosquitoes and Malaria*. Report of the Jubilee International Colloquium, Papua New Guinea Institute of Medical Research, Madang.

Buse K, Walt G. 2002. Globalisation and multilaterial public-private health partnerships: Issues for health policy. In: Lee K, Bruce K, Fustukian S, eds. *Health Policy in a Globalising World*. Cambridge, UK: Cambridge University Press. Pp. 41–62.

CDC (Centers for Disease Control and Prevention). 1999. Outbreaks of *Shigella sonnei* infection associated with eating fresh parsley—United States and Canada, July–August 1998. *MMWR* 48(14):285–290.

CDC. 2005. *Map: World Distribution of Dengue* [Online]. Available: http://www.cdc.gov/ncidod/dvbid/dengue/map-distribution-2005.htm [accessed October 18, 2005].

CDC. 2005a. *Map: Yellow Fever Endemic Zones in the Americas* [Online]. Available: http://www2.ncid.cdc.gov/travel/yb/utils/ybGet.asp?section=dis&obj=yellowfever.htm [accessed October 18, 2005].

CDC. 2005b. *Map: Yellow Fever Endemic Zones in Africa* [Online]. Available: http://www2.ncid.cdc.gov/travel/yb/utils/ybGet.asp?section=dis&obj=yellowfever.htm [accessed October 18, 2005].

Cetron M. 2002 (April 16). *The World and Its Moving Parts*. Presentation at the Institute of Medicine Workshop on the Impact of Globalization on Infectious Disease Emergence and Control: Exploring the Consequences and Opportunities, Washington, D.C. Institute of Medicine Forum on Emerging Infections.

Cleghorn F. 2002 (April 16). *Considering the Resources and Capacity for the Response*. Presentation at the Institute of Medicine Workshop on the Impact of Globalization on Infectious Disease Emergence and Control: Exploring the Consequences and Opportunities, Washington, D.C. Institute of Medicine Forum on Emerging Infections.

Corber S. 2002 (April 16). *Response to the Shifting Trends*. Presentation at the Institute of Medicine Workshop on the Impact of Globalization on Infectious Disease Emergence and Control: Exploring the Consequences and Opportunities, Washington, D.C. Institute of Medicine Forum on Emerging Infections.

Dragsted UB, Bauer J, Poulsen S, Askgaard D, Andersen AB, Lundgren JD. 1999. Epidemiology of tuberculosis in HIV-infected patients in Denmark. *Scand J Infect Dis* 31(1): 57–61.

El Alamy MA, Cline BL. 1997. Prevalence and intensity of *Schistosoma haematobium* and *S. mansoni* infection in Qalyub, Egypt. *Am J Trop Med Hyg* 26(3):470–472.

Friedman TL. 2000. *The Lexus and the Olive Tree: Understanding Globalization*. New York: Anchor Books.

Gordon D. 2002 (April 16). *The Global Infectious Disease Threat*. Presentation at the Institute of Medicine Workshop on the Impact of Globalization on Infectious Disease Emergence and Control: Exploring the Consequences and Opportunities, Washington, D.C. Institute of Medicine Forum on Emerging Infections.

Grondin D. 2002 (April 16). *Global Migration and Infectious Diseases*. Presentation at the Institute of Medicine Workshop on the Impact of Globalization on Infectious Disease Emergence and Control: Exploring the Consequences and Opportunities, Washington, D.C. Institute of Medicine Forum on Emerging Infections.

Gryseels B, Stelma FF, Talla I, van Dam GJ, Polman K, Sow S, Diaw M, Sturrock RF, Doehring-Schwerdtfeger E, Kardorff R. 1994. Epidemiology, immunology and chemotherapy of *Schistosoma mansoni* infections in a recently exposed community in Senegal. *Trop Geogr Med* 46:(4):209–219.

Hackett LW. 1937. *Malaria in Europe: An Ecological Study*. London, England: Oxford University Press. p. 226.

Hay SI, Cox J, Rogers DJ, Randolph SE, Stem DI, Shanks GD, Myers MF, Snow RW. 2002. Climate change and the resurgence of malaria in the East African highlands. *Nature* 415(6874):905–909.

IOM (Institute of Medicine). 2005. *The Threat of Pandemic Influenza: Are We Ready?* Washington, D.C: The National Academies Press.

Kimball AM. 2002 (April 16). *Considering the Resources and Capacity for Response*. Presentation at the Institute of Medicine Workshop on the Impact of Globalization on Infectious Disease Emergence and Control: Exploring the Consequences and Opportunities, Washington, D.C. Institute of Medicine Forum on Emerging Infections.

Leaning J. 2002 (April 16). *Health, Human Rights, and Humanitarian Assistance: The Medical and Public Health Response to Crises and Disasters*. Presentation at the Institute of Medicine Workshop on the Impact of Globalization on Infectious Disease Emergence and Control: Exploring the Consequences and Opportunities, Washington, D.C. Institute of Medicine Forum on Emerging Infections.

LeDuc J. 2002 (April 17). *The Global Application of Tools, Technology, and Knowledge to Counter the Consequences of Infectious Diseases: A Discussion of Priorities and Options*. Presentation at the Institute of Medicine Workshop on the Impact of Globalization on Infectious Disease Emergence and Control: Exploring the Consequences and Opportunities, Washington, D.C. Institute of Medicine Forum on Emerging Infections.

Lee K, Dodson R. 2000. Globalization and cholera: Implications for global governance. *Global Governance* 6(2):213–236.

Mayer J. 2002 (April 16). *Changing Vector Ecologies: Political Geographic Perspectives*. Presentation at the Institute of Medicine Workshop on the Impact of Globalization on Infectious Disease Emergence and Control: Exploring the Consequences and Opportunities, Washington, D.C. Institute of Medicine Forum on Emerging Infections.

NIC (National Intelligence Council). 2001. *Global Trends 2015*. [Online]. Available: http://www.cia.gov/cia/publications/globaltrends2015/ [accessed January 24, 2005].

Parfit M, Kasmauski K. 1998. Human migration. *National Geographic* 194(4):6–35.

Patz J. 2002 (April 16). *Invited Discussion: Considering the Resources and Capacity for Response.* Presentation at the Institute of Medicine Workshop on the Impact of Globalization on Infectious Disease Emergence and Control: Exploring the Consequences and Opportunities, Washington, D.C. Institute of Medicine Forum on Emerging Infections.

Rieder HL, Zellweger J-P, Raviglione MC, Keizer ST, Migliori GB. 1994. Tuberculosis Control in Europe and International Migration. Report of a Working Group. *Eur Respir J* 7(8):1545–1553.

Rogers DJ, Randolph SE. 2000. The global spread of malaria in a future, warmer world. *Science* 289(5485):1763–1766.

Sassen S. 1998. *Globalization and Its Discontents.* New York: New Press.

Silva IA, Nyland JF, Gorman A, Perisse A, Ventura AM, Santos EC, Souza JM, Burek CL, Rose NR, Silbergeld EK. 2004. Mercury exposure, malaria, and serum antinuclear/antinucleolar antibodies in Amazon populations in Brazil: A cross-sectional study. *Environmental Health* 3(1):11.

Soros G. 2002. *George Soros on Globalization.* New York: Public Affairs.

Widdus R. 2002 (April 17). *Partnering for Success: The Role of Private-Public Sector Collaboration.* Presentation at the Institute of Medicine Workshop on the Impact of Globalization on Infectious Disease Emergence and Control: Exploring the Consequences and Opportunities, Washington, D.C. Institute of Medicine Forum on Emerging Infections.

Wilson M. 2002 (April 16). *Invited Discussion: A Response to the Shifting Trends.* Presentation at the Institute of Medicine Workshop on the Impact of Globalization on Infectious Disease Emergence and Control: Exploring the Consequences and Opportunities, Washington, D.C. Institute of Medicine Forum on Emerging Infections.

2

Examining the Consequences:
A Changing Landscape

From the transcontinental movement of people to the global flow of capital, the multitude of complex, interacting phenomena described in Chapter 1 will, if left unchecked, continue to shape the global landscape in dramatic and unpredictable ways. This chapter provides a summary of the workshop presentations and discussions focused on some of the ways in which the global landscape is already changing or expected to change in ways that could cause or exacerbate the emergence and global spread of infectious diseases.

Most notably, the growing demographic and economic divides between rich and poor countries, combined with increasing levels of access to information even in the remotest corners of the world, are expected to fuel widespread discontent, armed conflict, and the massive displacement of people, the public health consequences of which are often disastrous. Refugee populations are among the most vulnerable to emerging and reemerging infectious diseases. Summarized here are the presentations and discussions pertaining to these growing economic and demographic gaps, the consequences of armed conflict for public health, and the need for improved screening and surveillance of mobile populations—not just war-displaced refugees, but also all migrant populations.

The surveillance of mobile populations is only one of several types of surveillance urgently in need of development or revamping. As the transcontinental movement of food and commodities has increased, so, too, has the need for improved trade- and food-related surveillance; discussion of this topic is also included here. (Opportunities and obstacles with regard to the development of a general global infectious disease surveillance system are discussed in Chapter 3.)

Another notable feature of the changing global landscape is the increased perceived and actual threat of bioterrorism, particularly in the United States. In response, the Bush Administration has proposed an unprecedented amount of public health funding—approximately $6 billion—for defense against bioterrorism (biodefense). These funds are expected to have both direct and indirect benefits for the prevention and control of emerging and reemerging infectious diseases in general, whether intentionally or naturally introduced, by strengthening the public health community's ability to make constructive changes in a way never before possible. The discussion of this topic is summarized here as well. (Presentations and discussions pertaining to increased spending on international health in general, including funds that are not necessarily U.S. biodefense–related, are summarized in Chapter 4.)

Finally, this chapter includes summaries of regional case studies presented by representatives of Russia and the European Union. Both provide important insights into the impact of globalization on public health in parts of the developed world outside of the United States. In the case of Russia, the collapse of the cold war political system has led to widespread social and public health problems manifested in multiple ways, most notably a rise in the numbers of people with HIV/AIDS and multidrug-resistant tuberculosis (TB). The current situation illustrates how even an educated population and a plenitude of natural resources cannot guarantee good public health if political and other leaders do not consider health a priority.

The situation in the European Union, on the other hand, may provide a useful model for understanding how the public health impacts of the movement of capital, resources, and people across former political boundaries can be managed. It is unclear, however, whether the European model can actually be applied to other, less unified areas of the world. Moreover, despite its successes, the region is still experiencing serious problems with respect to emerging infectious diseases, for example, among migrant populations.

ECONOMIC GAPS, GLOBAL DISCONTENT, COMMUNAL CONFLICT, AND FORCED MIGRATION[1]

Globalizing forces are expected to increase and exacerbate already tense relationships between rich and poor countries, as has been witnessed in the

---

[1]This section is based on the workshop presentations by Gordon (2002), Leaning (2002), and LeDuc (2002).

intense international debate regarding intellectual property rights and the affordability of antiretroviral agents. A National Intelligence Council report (NIC, 2000) predicts that over the next 15 years, this international economic divergence will probably continue. Although developed countries and some developing countries will continue to enjoy high rates of economic growth, the rates in most developing countries will be very stunted. The situation will be exacerbated by the fact that infectious diseases, particularly HIV/AIDS, will continue to depress economic growth in the hardest-hit countries by as much as one percent of their gross domestic product (GDP) per year; over the course of many years, the impact of this will be huge.

Recent massive changes in international trade law are fueling a great deal of discomfort and unhappiness in the developing world, and poorer countries are already pressing harder to gain access to markets in the developed world. One of the most recent, conspicuous changes in international trade fora is the strengthening voice of developing countries. It is no accident that the current round of multilateral trade negotiations has explicitly been named the "Development Round," to reflect the growing importance of trade to the developing world. The debate over access to antiretroviral drugs for the treatment of HIV infection suggests that these kinds of issues are likely to become increasingly common points of tension in future trade negotiations.

Moreover, the tremendous advances and expansions in communication that are being made possible by today's technology have provided many, although not all, parts of the world with unprecedented access to television. People around the world know how everybody else is living. Greater knowledge and a changing perception of the increasing social and economic disparities between rich and poor countries will likely continue to fuel widespread antiglobalist sentiments and frustration. For some, knowing that they are not living to the same standard as others is a source of great discontent.

In many parts of the world, governance is not strong enough to handle the daunting pressure on states' capacities to adjust to these global shifts in trade, communication, and perception. A relationship with the people, the capacity to be flexible in times of community distress, and the ability to respond to the ongoing resistance posed by the opposition party all require a sophistication and capacity that many of these countries lack. The pressure to respond creates a greater propensity to state failure. From Zimbabwe to Venezuela, this fragility of government in the face of globalization must be kept in mind. State collapse provides the opportunity for an influx of nonstate actors. The regional instability that often ensues increases the risk of armed conflict, which in turn leads to the massive displacement of people and humanitarian and public health crises.

Communal Conflicts and Small Arms

Several think tanks worldwide have investigated the issue of small-arms availability. They have examined the magnitude of the problem, the prevalence and production of small arms, the trade routes used, the amount of money circulating in the trade, impacts in countries where the arms are used, and the major players.

The majority of wars are waged with small arms.[2] Most of these conflicts are communally based fights between racial, ethnic, tribal, or language groups within larger populations. Although local, these wars are aggravated by regional and global factors, including poor leadership, underlying socioeconomic conditions, and communications with the diaspora. Once ignited, these conflicts tend to be long-lived, generally lasting at least 10 years. Some are well into their thirtieth year.

Most populations engaged in communal conflicts suffer from irresponsible or malignant leadership, and such conflicts occur in collapsing or failing states where human rights abuses are rampant. Most of the nonstate actors who wage such wars or who cause complex humanitarian emergencies (as the public health community refers to them) are not part of the established power structure. Rather, they tend to be informal armies, militias, and rebels who are not completely contained by a chain of command and typically are unconcerned about international humanitarian law. Their strategy is to target civilians by committing acts of terror or ethnic cleansing or by capturing land and forcing populations to flee. They follow this strategy for two principal reasons: they have not been educated in other strategies, and they have easy access to small arms, the only weapons available to them.

The definition of a small arm is constantly evolving, but essentially encompasses any weapon that can be used by one to three people, including submachine guns and assault rifles, mounted grenade launchers, and portable antiaircraft missiles and missile launchers. Of all the key underlying conditions that promote or sustain conflict—poverty, arms availability, communal tensions, and state failure—arms availability is the most directly affected by globalization.

---

[2]Major recent exceptions include the first Gulf War, which involved massive arms used by a first-world power, the United States, and its allies; Kosovo, which involved NATO (North Atlantic Treaty Organization) forces (i.e., not the Kosovo Liberation Army and Serbian forces that were at work in 1998–1999, which used small arms); Ethiopia and Eritrea, where in the 1990s a massive conventional war with large heavy weapons killed 80,000 to 100,000 people; and, most recently but subsequent to this workshop, the Iraq War.

Small arms can be purchased from a thriving global market that includes about $3–6 billion in legal sales and $2–10 billion in illegal sales annually. There are more than 500 million small-arms weapons in circulation—one for every 12 people on earth. About a third of a million people die each year from wounds caused by the small arms used in war; another 200,000 people die each year from wounds caused by handguns during peacetime.

Legal transfer represents a major share of the small-arms trade, one that could be influenced by U.S. policy. Policy changes that affected the legal market would also affect the "gray" market, where sales are possibly legal but either secret or unauthorized in small-arms trade laws. The illegal black market, however, cannot even be monitored because it takes place in remote, inaccessible, or highly dangerous areas and remains overlooked because of corruption.

Enormous humanitarian impacts result from the prevalence of these weapons in societies that are already disintegrating because of state collapse and the encroachment of rebel forces operating outside the rule of law. In Afghanistan, for example, virtually every male over the age of nine possesses an AK-47 assault rifle. It can be terrifying to live in a society where the availability of small arms disrupts traditional modes of conflict resolution. Traditionally, for example, if a man's cow were stolen, he might kill one of the thief's animals with his knife. Or if a man's woman were insulted, he might attack someone in the suspect's family with a long-bore, single-shot rifle. The situation is quite different today, with grenades, land mines, and assault rifles being at everyone's disposal, and is exacerbated by the escalating cycle of reprisal and action. Many people living in such areas (e.g., Somalia and Sudan) say the situation is out of control.

In the postconflict setting, disarmament of a population in which the presence of small arms is so diffuse and pervasive is politically daunting. The persistence of the weapons retards the transition to work, deters investors from the developed world, and leads to the rise of criminal elements, as is currently happening, for example, in Liberia and Sierra Leone.

Forced Migration

Communal conflicts are characterized by the massive dislocation of populations and extensive destruction of infrastructure. An estimated 50 million people worldwide are forcibly displaced from their homes each year; this displaced population includes migrants who move regularly to find work and refugees who flee to a foreign country to escape danger. The United States alone receives an average of 90,000 refugees annually. Refugee populations are among the most vulnerable to emerging infectious diseases, even more so than migrants (see Chapter 1). For example, on the basis of preliminary data from a 2000 International Organization for Migration assessment of the health of more than 76,000 mobile people (44.7 percent migrants, 55.3 percent refugees), refugees are more likely than migrants to be HIV-positive (representing 65 percent of HIV-positive individuals in the database) (Grondin, 2002).

The breakdown of public health systems and the public sector generally in areas that are experiencing war or receiving migrants can be profound. In many war-torn areas, public health systems are so severely affected that they do not have the capacity to provide adequate services. The rates of death and disease in Afghanistan, for example, are among the highest in the world. The maternal mortality rate in Afghanistan is on the order of 1,700 maternal deaths per 10,000 live births—close to what one would expect if there were no health care at all. Fully 25 percent of children in Afghanistan die before the age of five years, and about 20 percent before their first birthday. The country is experiencing a breakdown at all levels of health care, and immunization is almost nonexistent. Although there is little concern about a mass epidemic in Afghanistan since the country is not densely populated, its dire situation illustrates the devastating effects war can have on public health.

The situation is often exacerbated by the fact that forced migration can escalate or precipitate further conflict. This occurs especially in regional and host settings in Africa and Central Asia where massive influxes of people fleeing one war feed into a local diaspora that is also part of an unwanted ethnic group in the host country. For example, Georgia, Armenia, Afghanistan, and the surrounding countries are sites of regional tumult where migrants move from one area of distress and sow another in their host country. Because the receiving countries are typically poor and already border the war-torn areas, the refugees tax the host governments even further.

Workshop participants noted that refugees are not the only people who serve as infectious disease vectors during wartime. Peacekeepers do so as well. This is especially true for HIV/AIDS, as the parallel progression of the HIV/AIDS epidemic and the peacekeeper movement in many parts of Africa illustrates. Kosovo may be experiencing the beginning of a similar war-related HIV/AIDS epidemic. Before the war in Kosovo and the introduction of peacekeepers, not a single case of HIV/AIDS was known in the area, according to Kosovo's Institute of Public Health. Since the arrival of peacekeepers, however, the incidence of HIV/AIDS has been increasing.

Peacekeepers can be disease vectors for a variety of reasons. Peacekeeping soldiers generally arrive in areas in large numbers, more often engage in sexual activity than does the general population, and frequently behave in a predatory manner; these behaviors among soldiers have been witnessed for centuries. Moreover, a number of studies have shown that when peacekeepers move into an area, the prevalence of HIV/AIDS increases significantly, not only in the host country but in the adjoining countries as well, because of the sex trade. Sex workers flock to where the peacekeepers are located, moving back and forth across borders and spreading disease. In addition, biological evidence suggests that the infectivity rate is highest during the early phases of HIV infection, when the viral load is very high; therefore, newly infected soldiers with many sexual partners initiate spirals of disease propagation.

One participant asked whether, when peacekeeping forces are assembled, deferred compensation is ever considered as a means of constraining the social impact of the economic imbalance between the peacekeeping forces and the general population, especially since this economic imbalance is what drives the sex trade. For example, the much higher per diem of the United Nations Transitional Authority in Cambodia relative to the average daily wage of Cambodians led to an explosion of the prostitution industry in that country and the movement of HIV into Cambodia from Vietnam. In response to this question, a participant stated that, although a great deal of attention is being focused on the prevalence of HIV infection among peacekeeping forces, the issue is very politically charged. Many countries that provide peacekeeping forces do so because they receive a small amount of money from the United Nations to augment their military budgets; these countries are too poor to provide treatment for their soldiers and thus refuse to have them tested for HIV. Those countries that do test their forces and treat their HIV-positive soldiers, including Great Britain, the United States, Canada, and some western European countries, are less likely to provide forces for peacekeeping missions.

Another participant pointed out that the economic imbalance existing in war-torn areas is not limited to peacekeepers. The United Nations and other nongovernmental organizations and bilateral agencies pay their international staff five to 20 times more than is customary in the local economy, creating massive economic distortion. Anyone who can speak English or the most common language in the given location is drawn from the local labor market, a talent drain that can take years to redress. This is happening in the Balkans, for example, as well as in Afghanistan, and has occurred in the past in many parts of Africa, including Angola and Sudan. A participant suggested that perhaps the United Nations could address this issue if and when the humanitarian community becomes more organized.

SURVEILLANCE OF MOBILE POPULATIONS[3]

The incidence rates of TB and multidrug-resistant TB in migrant populations (see Chapter 1) illustrate the tremendous risk of acquiring and

---

[3]This section is based on the workshop presentations by Barry (2002), Cetron (2002), Grondin (2002), and LeDuc (2002).

transmitting infectious diseases among mobile populations, especially those originating in poor countries with a high prevalence of disease. Preventing and controlling the emergence and spread of TB and other infectious diseases among mobile populations will require that gaps in public health infrastructure among countries be bridged, particularly gaps between countries that generate and receive migrants. Although mobility, technologies, and economies may no longer be constrained by borders, political boundaries still limit public health infrastructure. This is perhaps nowhere more evident than in the surveillance of mobile populations. There is an urgent need to shift away from traditionally fragmented provincial, state, or local health department–based surveillance infrastructures toward a more global approach to data acquisition and information sharing.

At the same time, the need for a new, borderless approach to managing the health of mobile populations should not detract from the continuing need for strong domestic medical training programs. In particular, the medical staff in receiving countries, including the United States, need to be better trained to treat migrants. Physicians should be able to recognize and treat those infectious diseases, such as multidrug-resistant TB, that are most likely to affect migrants.

Migrant Screening Criteria

The procedures used to screen mobile populations vary among countries. Countries that have traditionally received large numbers of migrants—including the United States, Australia, Canada, and New Zealand—conduct prearrival medical screening for migrants with active and infective TB and mandatory testing for HIV. The criteria used to determine who will be screened before arrival include the incidence rates of specific infectious diseases in the country of origin, the category of the applicant (e.g., refugee vs. migrant), and the individual's occupation and expected length of stay in the receiving country. European and other countries with more recent immigration histories rely on postarrival screening, as demanded by work permits or refugee immigration statutes.

Prearrival screening may appear to be the ideal model for preventing the importation of TB and other infectious diseases. In reality, however, it is truly effective only in the case of well-organized, well-managed, and well-planned migration movements; it could not possibly be used to manage today's global mobile population. Moreover, prearrival screening based on immigration status is not necessarily the most effective way to manage migrant health. According to the above-mentioned 2000 International Organization for Migration assessment of the health of mobile people, in contrast with the case of HIV, the incidence of TB was about eight percent higher among migrants than among refugees (Grondin, 2002). This finding is of note, given that certain classes of migrants, such as long-term visitors in the United States, are usually excluded from the screening requirements. A 2001 study of TB incidence in Tarrant County, Texas, for example, found that nonimmigrant, long-term visitors had a higher rate of TB and multidrug-resistant TB than immigrants (Weis et al., 2001). In this light, there is a need to revisit migration health surveillance programs targeting only refugees or permanent residents.

Refugee health in particular is complicated by the inability to track refugee departures, transit times, and arrivals accurately, making it difficult both to acquire prescreening information and to transmit that information to government resettlement programs before refugees report for postarrival screening. Moreover, in many countries the multidrug-resistant TB detection rate from the screening of migrants is suboptimal at best, and basic supervision of sputum collection procedures is often lacking. In some developed countries, applicants are told to conduct sputum testing at home, without proper supervision. In addition, patients with active TB can have smear-negative sputa if they are being treated.

Despite the difficulties of screening mobile populations, many programs are undergoing significant changes that will likely have positive effects on the health of these populations.

- The International Organization for Migration is sponsoring the development of a pilot electronic notification system that will receive health screening data and provide swift electronic notification of all patients with infectious smear-positive (class A) TB, as well as those who are smear negative but still require follow-up and those with latent TB infection (LTBI) who require prophylactic follow-up.

- A recent Institute of Medicine report (IOM, 2000) called for the institution of procedures for the screening of migrants with LTBI before they leave their home country, an enormous task extending beyond traditional entry requirements. However, with the realization that reliable partners in other countries are capable of much more sophisticated predeparture management, more challenging goals are being set. This is true not just for patients with TB, but also for those with other infectious diseases. Before departure, for example, African refugees are treated with antimalarial agents in an effort to relieve some of the extra burden on countries that cannot readily recognize or diagnose malaria.

- Because sputum smears can be converted so readily, efforts are under way to develop more sensitive and appropriate screening algorithms, including culture-based approaches, polymerase chain reaction–based methods, and the addition of adjuvants to sputum for testing purposes.

Workshop participants offered several additional ideas for effecting positive change. One participant suggested that recent dramatic discussion in the media about calls from some political leaders to abolish the Immigration and Naturalization Service (INS)[4] indicated an opportunity to work toward making changes in that agency to better address the migrant and refugee health issues described above. Another proposed that recent advances in telemedicine may provide innovative opportunities for migrant health screening. Finally, as discussed earlier, it was emphasized that U.S. health care providers need to be better informed and prepared to deal with the health needs of mobile populations. To this end, a health education curriculum addressing migrants/refugees should perhaps be established for U.S. physicians.

One participant expressed concern that there is no uniform procedure for refugee screening and that, currently, refugees can be prescreened up to a year before entering the United States. The suggestion was made that the prescreening interval be shortened to less than one year. In response, it was noted that technical instructions for overseas medical screening of refugee populations are being rewritten to shorten the duration from one year to 6 months.

Another participant suggested that a centralized website for geographic surveillance of refugee populations be established. In response, it was noted that GeoSentinel, a global network of 22 travel/tropical medicine clinics (14 in the United States and eight in other countries) that monitor the health status of mobile populations, has increasingly focused on refugee health clinics. When the network was established in 1996, its initial emphasis was on collecting disease- or syndrome-specific diagnoses on returning travelers, immigrants, and foreign visitors (Freedman et al., 1999). The network now includes about 25 refugee health clinics as well. There is some concern, however, that GeoSentinel may not be comprehensive since (with variation from one site to another) refugees are not required to visit a refugee (or travel) clinic, are very broadly dispersed, and are also unlikely to see any local provider (Cetron, 2002). Depending on how a country spends its local resources for refugee health, national health departments may or may not be able to accommodate refugee health care, which tends to be distributed mainly among local providers, not refugee clinics. This is true even though GeoSentinel clinics are not required to be based in national health departments and can be in the private sector. Another concern regarding GeoSentinel is that its website—which posts surveillance data for tourist, refugee, and immigrant movements—needs to be further developed and

---

[4]The INS ceased to exist on November 25, 2002, when the last of its functions were transferred to the new Department of Homeland Security.

better surveillance information needs to be gathered and made more readily available (Cetron, 2002).

Recommendations of the International Organization for Migration for Improved TB Screening of Mobile Populations

Despite the obvious challenges, improved TB control programs for mobile populations are possible. Such programs will need to involve both predeparture screening in countries of origin and postarrival screening in receiving countries. The greatest challenge is probably faced by policy makers and researchers; this is true not only for TB, but also for HIV/AIDS and other infectious diseases. The International Organization for Migration has made the following recommendations for TB control programs:

- Even in the country of origin, it is essential that sputum collection be supervised, laboratory personnel be comprehensively trained, a consistent system of quality control and quality assurance be implemented, and complete treatment be conducted under observation (i.e., using directly observed therapy).
- Countries that receive migrants must share information and public health tools with and provide feedback to countries of origin.
- Faster, more efficient information systems are needed for communication between countries of origin and receiving countries.
- Existing surveillance systems must be strengthened, and an international surveillance system linking countries of origin and host countries must be implemented.
- A public health justification for providing all migrants access to health care, particularly those who do not have legal status, must be formulated.
- Vulnerability to infection must be reduced by improving the living conditions of migrant populations.
- Disease prevention strategies for mobile populations must be developed to decrease stigmatization and discrimination within both host countries and receiving local communities.

One of the most important issues with regard to screening for TB is the need to formulate screening criteria that are replicable, reliable, and affordable in terms of laboratory support. For example, even individuals who have positive skin tests but do not develop active TB may benefit from prophylactic therapy, and even those who test negative may still be infected and require ongoing treatment.

FOODBORNE AND TRADE-RELATED
INFECTIOUS DISEASE SURVEILLANCE[5]

It may appear that foodborne infectious disease outbreaks with a domestic origin are a greater problem than those originating from imported products, at least in the United States (see Chapter 1). However, workshop participants noted that the relatively few documented examples of infectious disease outbreaks resulting from the importation of contaminated food may reflect inadequate surveillance and detection more than the actual incidence of disease. Like population surveillance, global food surveillance—and surveillance of trade-related infectious disease in general[6] —is lacking in capacity and requires major improvement. This is the case even though international trade in agricultural products has been steadily increasing over the last 30 years, to the point where in 2000, trade in fruit and vegetables amounted to $160 billion; that in meat and meat products to $90 billion; and that in dairy products, eggs, and live animals to $60 billion. Even if foodborne infectious disease outbreaks do not occur more often than the numbers that have been recorded, the potential for such outbreaks is undoubtedly on the rise.

One of the main challenges associated with trade-related infectious disease surveillance is that subsequent epidemiological investigations are necessary to link detected outbreaks or occurrences of infectious diseases to trade. The epidemiological investigation surrounding the cyclosporiasis outbreaks in North America (see Chapter 1) was exemplary, mainly because the microbe, a fairly new agent, stimulated a great deal of exciting scientific discovery. If these outbreaks had been caused by something as common and well known as *Salmonella*, the epidemiological details would probably not have been nearly as elegant. Another major challenge to the implementation of effective surveillance of trade-related infectious disease

---

[5]This section is based on the workshop presentations by Acheson (2002), Corber (2002), and Kimball (2002).

[6]During their investigations of the relationship between trade and infectious diseases over the past 5 years, University of Washington researchers, in collaboration with Asia-Pacific Economic Cooperation, the World Trade Organization, and the World Health Organization, have identified three working definitions of trade-related infectious diseases: (1) infectious diseases whose emergence is hastened by the ecological pressures of scaling up production to meet the demands of international markets (some people, however, question whether scaling up is really the cause of the proliferation of a potential human pathogen, such as new variant Jakob-Creutzfeldt disease, and consider this definition a hypothetical construct useful only for the examination of plausible mechanisms); (2) infectious diseases whose transmission is broadened through the transportation or trading of goods (e.g., the broad geographic dissemination of trade-based infections); and (3) an infectious disease that has a large economic impact in terms of trade disruption.

is that insufficient trade-related information is entered into surveillance system databases to allow the early detection of such events.

Although the World Health Organization (WHO) and the World Trade Organization (WTO) operate entirely differently, both play a role in establishing and monitoring regulations and rules that govern how food and other products are kept safe in the international marketplace. WHO, a 192-member specialized agency of the United Nations whose primary mandate is to improve health, administers the International Health Regulations (see Chapter 4) and the *Codex Alimentarius*, which sets food standards. WTO, a smaller agency that deals with trade-related issues, comprises multiple working groups. Some of the more pertinent of these working groups are Trade-Related Aspects of Intellectual Property Rights (TRIPS), Sanitary and Phytosanitary Measures (SPS), and Technical Barriers to Trade (TBT).

Both WHO and WTO have recently made efforts to improve trade-related infectious disease surveillance on a global scale. For example, WHO has diversified its sources of reporting and can now accept reports from informal sources as well as ministries of health. As another example, WTO has implemented an urgent-measures reporting system, which obliges member countries to report when they restrict imports because of infectious diseases; as a result, the rates of reporting of import restrictions increased from 1996 to 2001. Most of the restrictions on food and agricultural products were associated with concerns regarding animal health (42 percent) and food safety (38 percent); foot-and-mouth disease accounted for 36 percent of the restrictions, and bovine spongiform encephalopathy for 21 percent.

The stated priorities of various other regional working groups, such as Asia-Pacific Economic Cooperation (APEC), reflect an increasing concern with trade-related infectious diseases. APEC leaders identified infectious disease surveillance as a priority issue when they met in Shanghai, China, in 2001 and are in the process of creating a network of networks to enhance the regional capacity for infectious disease surveillance throughout the Pacific. The APEC strategy calls for innovative uses of web-based reporting systems among APEC countries and the use of electronic reporting systems already developed by the countries themselves. Other regional efforts include the European Union's creation of a laboratory-based network for surveillance for enteric disease and Legionnaires' disease, and the Association of Southeast Asian Nations' syndromic surveillance system for early warnings of disease clusters. In light of APEC's efforts, one participant suggested that the public health community may be lagging in appreciating the importance of trade-related infectious disease surveillance.

Recent efforts to improve food surveillance in particular include the U.S. Department of Agriculture's (USDA) involvement in globalizing food safety by examining inspection processes in other countries, helping others meet USDA requirements, and participating in policy decisions in many collaborative inspector training programs. USDA does not, however, actually conduct food safety inspections in other countries.

Despite steps being taken WHO, WTO, APEC, USDA, and other organizations, several major challenges to improving global trade-related infectious disease surveillance remain, and most of these are due to the disjointed efforts of different agencies or geographic regions. For example, WTO and WHO need to integrate their information and regulatory systems—a major challenge, as the two organizations operate quite differently. In addition, although regional trading blocks, such as Mercosur in South America (involving Argentina, Brazil, Paraguay, and Uruguay), are moving forward, they are doing so in very diverse ways, depending on the region. Finally, there is great variation among countries and regions in the strengths and capacities of the laboratory-based infrastructure for epidemiological surveillance, a key component of trade-related infectious disease surveillance. A weak laboratory capacity affects not only infectious disease surveillance, but also the ability to make scientifically informed decisions about whether trade should be disrupted on the basis of the occurrence of an epidemic disease.

INCREASED BIODEFENSE SPENDING: OPPORTUNITIES AND CONCERNS[7]

Throughout the workshop, discussion focused on the unprecedented amount of available or promised federal funds for biodefense prompted by the terrorist attacks of September 11, 2001, and the subsequent mailing of anthrax spore–laden letters. The approximately $6 billion in funding committed to biodefense affords a significant opportunity to strengthen the capacity of the United States to contribute to the control and management of global emerging infectious disease threats, but it also raises many concerns regarding the use of the funds.

Use of Funding for Biodefense in the Context of Emerging and Reemerging Infectious Diseases

One of the greatest challenges posed by the new funding for biodefense is how to use this vast amount of resources within the context of emerging

---

[7]This section is based on the workshop presentations by Cash (2002), Corber (2002), Gardner (2002), Heyman (2002), Kurth (2002), Leaning (2002), LeDuc (2002), and Miller (2002).

and reemerging infectious diseases. After all, bioterrorism represents only one end of a spectrum of infectious disease threats, and category A diseases and agents are not the only potential bioterrorist weapons. A national or global public health system with the capacity to respond quickly and effectively to intentionally introduced infectious disease threats would also likely have the capacity to respond to naturally occurring infectious disease threats. Most of the priorities for capacity building are the same for both types of threat. In fact, one could argue that the problems of bioterrorism cannot be solved until the problems of infectious diseases generally are solved.

For example, one of the key priorities for action identified during the workshop is strengthening linkages between clinical medicine and public health, a measure that would have profound benefits for both biodefense and the prevention and control of infectious diseases in general. As one participant noted, it was an alert clinician in southern Florida who recognized the index case in the anthrax attack in that state. Yet at present, only a relatively small pool of professionals have these skills. The professional and training needs required to bridge this gap are immense (see Chapter 3).

As another example, communication was probably the most challenging aspect of the response to the anthrax attacks, pointing to the urgent need for improved communication in the global infectious disease surveillance and response system. Improved communication would also benefit both biodefense and the prevention and control of naturally introduced infectious diseases. (For further discussion of surveillance, see the section on surveillance earlier in this chapter and the section on global surveillance in Chapter 3.)

About a third of the new funds for biodefense is being dedicated to basic research, including the development of new platform technologies for diagnosis, surveillance, and treatment, which should be broadly applicable to a wide range of infectious diseases. Some of the funds allocated to basic research will be directed specifically toward developing a better understanding of the innate immune system, which again is fundamentally important in the fight against any infectious disease. Because there are so many potential bioterrorist agents, it is impossible to develop a specific vaccine or therapy for each, and money spent on basic vaccine and antibiotic research for the purposes of strengthening biodefense is expected to have a major beneficial impact on the effort to control other, nonbioterrorist infectious threats as well. Clearly, strengthening basic research in the name of biodefense will likely yield numerous overall benefits in the long run. One workshop participant referred to these secondary effects of biodefense spending as the "spillover effect."

Two examples of this spillover effect are greater access to TB treatment and improved health care for the elderly. At present, TB treatment is helping less than 30 percent of the world's TB patients; the increased global investments in health care infrastructure made in the name of biodefense could expand the reach of these and other programs to the remainder of the populace. The new funding for biodefense could also indirectly improve access to health care for the elderly, a growing portion of the world's population that places a heavy demand on health care infrastructure. It is estimated that in 2025, 1.2 billion people worldwide will be over age 60. By 2050, that number will almost double in developed countries alone, and 80 percent of people over age 60 will be living in developing countries. New breakthroughs resulting from increased spending on biodefense not only may advance life-enhancing technologies, but also may lower the enormous costs of the health care required by this aging population. In developing countries, where the cost of medicines—whether quality drugs or counterfeits—may easily exceed the purchasing power of the people, these reduced costs may also increase the medicines' availability and use.

The new funds have the potential to affect public health not only in the United States but also throughout the world by providing opportunities for increased spending on foreign aid and the implementation of measures needed to improve public health and surveillance in developing countries. A workshop participant noted that this could occur in many ways. For example, the availability of the funding has elicited a strong call for the development of overseas surveillance networks of the type that would enhance the work of such groups as the U.S. Naval Medical Research Unit 3 (NAMRU-3) in Cairo, Egypt.

Finally, participants noted that the recent influx of money has motivated a number of individual players from around the world, including overseas units of the Centers for Disease Control and Prevention (CDC) and the U.S. Department of Defense, to convene for discussion and collaboration. This type of dialogue was crucial in the case of the anthrax attacks, as no single entity had all of the information necessary for a prompt, effective response. Communication and cooperation are vital components of any program for the global control of emerging and reemerging infectious diseases, whether the goal is to thwart potential bioterrorist attacks or to protect the general public health.

Warnings

Despite the optimism regarding the potential benefits of the new funding, some participants expressed concern that there is a limited time within which to answer this call to action, either domestically or internationally, and the world may never have this chance again. All parties involved must be committed to doing the best they can to rebuild systems across the board and around the world. Moreover, the health sector must communicate much better with its constituencies, both within the United States and worldwide. In the opinion of one participant, WHO has recently made an impressive investment in improving its communication capacity by hiring individuals who specialize not in health, but in effectively communicating messages to the masses. CDC and the overall health community need to take a cue from this effort, and the United States needs to do a better job of educating and informing policy makers and decision makers and ensuring that the opportunity to reach the widest possible audience is not missed.

The admonition was also expressed that although nearly $6 billion is being devoted to efforts to combat bioterrorism, biodefense does not necessarily have repercussions, either positive or negative, for other infectious disease threats. Indeed, only about one-fifth of the money for biodefense is budgeted for what might be considered the "classic" public health sector.

Moreover, it is unclear exactly how the funds will be spent, and there could even be a distorting effect from spending such large amounts so quickly. Even though some of the funding will go toward vaccines, antibiotics, and basic research through the National Institutes of Health, all of which are essential public health components, providing money for those efforts is not the same as adding desperately needed new staff positions to the public health system or strengthening surveillance activities. For example, although the enormous smallpox vaccine production effort will boost U.S. biodefense capabilities and make the nation's population safer, it cannot really be said to make anybody healthier since smallpox has already been eradicated. As another example, about 70 percent of the Egyptian population has schistosomiasis, but it is unclear how NAMRU-3 is going to benefit from U.S. biodefense efforts. In theory, then, funding for biodefense should be a great help in combating infectious diseases, but it remains unknown whether the money will actually be spent in a way that will aid the most people as efficiently and quickly as possible.

It should not be forgotten that the threat of bioterrorism is real and requires a targeted, focused, well-funded effort. Bioterrorism is, after all, the poor person's weapon of the future. In the early 1980s, it was asked whether everyone would eventually be able to have a personal computer. Today the question being asked is whether there will come a day when everyone will be able to have the desktop computer equivalent of a biological laboratory. Could teenage biological "hackers" unwittingly develop and accidentally release genetically modified organisms, with catastrophic results? Might they inadvertently develop the biological analog to the "Love Bug," which wreaked havoc on computers around the world? Might a suicide attacker log on to PriceLine.com and, for the price of a ticket, spread a virulent disease across the globe?

Although in October 2001 anthrax spores were not used as a weapon of mass destruction in terms of human lives lost, they were used as a weapon of mass disruption. The economic implications were great. The United States Postal Service spent more than $3 billion on upgrading security and reallocating workers, while the clean-up cost was more than $24 million at the Hart congressional office building complex; as of this writing, clean-up of the American Media Incorporated Building and the Brentwood postal facility has yet to be completed. If an infectious agent other than anthrax spores had been used, the effect could have been horrific in terms of both the number of lives lost and the psychological and economic ramifications. As it was, the response effort required the participation of thousands of people from the public health and law enforcement communities. Indeed, since September 11, 2001, law enforcement officials have responded to more than 8,000 incidents purportedly involving weapons of mass destruction. While most of these incidents were hoaxes, they have caused a tremendous drain on resources at a time when those resources are desperately needed to carry out the war on terrorism.

Although investigation of the anthrax attacks has consumed a tremendous number of person-hours and although the Federal Bureau of Investigation, working closely with health officials, has done an extraordinary job, what is known about the attacks is still less than what is unknown, according to one participant. The Ames strain of *Bacillus anthracis* used in the attacks is distributed throughout the world, making it difficult to track down a potential source. In addition, although the spores were coated with silica, which neither Russia nor the United States has used in its domestic programs, this is not necessarily a very helpful clue given the accessibility of modern biochemical components and techniques. Thus the country still does not know whether the source of the anthrax spores was domestic or foreign. Nor is it known whether there is a connection between the person or persons responsible for the attacks and those responsible for the attacks of September 11. To make matters more difficult, the investigation is encumbered by a culture clash between law enforcement officials and scientists. The former prefer to move forward in a lockstep fashion, whereas the latter tend to ask more questions and engage in more discussion.

It is also important to note that this was not the first bioterrorist attack on the United States. The salmonella poisoning event that took place in Oregon in 1983 did not garner the attention it perhaps should have received. Bioterrorism was not on the radar screen at the time, and experts did not even realize the act was deliberate until a year after it occurred.

Furthermore, while preparing for future biodefense efforts and addressing bioterrorism-related issues, it is essential that policy makers, scientists, and others consider not only which biological weapons terrorists are developing to use against the United States and other countries, but also the underlying ways in which globalization is creating the distress and fury that cause them to do so. The political and social capacity to understand and address these underlying issues is essential.

Participants also cautioned that the flow of money to combat bioterrorism could disappear as quickly as it appeared. It is unclear whether funding of the current magnitude can be sustained over the long term, as it must be if it is to make a real difference in controlling either intentionally or naturally introduced infectious diseases. For example, although the recent budgetary changes may allow the establishment of several new staff positions in a single public health office, the positions may last only one or two years, depending on the sustainability of the funds.

In light of the issue of long-term sustainability, the need for clear communication is, again, paramount. A participant suggested that one of the basic priorities for action should be educating individuals and groups that are responsible for distributing the funds. It is critical for those in decision-making positions to understand how globalization increases the vulnerability not only of the developing world but also of the United States to infectious disease threats. Otherwise, the United States may find itself in the position of having seen the handwriting on the wall without having done anything about it. For example, the reintroduction of mosquito vectors worldwide and the resurgence of TB both illustrate the consequences of the complacency that results when the numbers of cases of a particular disease decrease and its visible manifestations disappear. When resources, attention, and capability are prematurely redirected, the world suffers long-term consequences. One possibility would be for the public health community to develop a congressional fellowship program similar to that of the American Association for the Advancement of Science. Public health congressional fellows could help draft policy and provide the knowledge base needed by legislators to make informed decisions.

Finally, several participants expressed concern that the new biodefense efforts are creating a serious capacity challenge in the United States and worldwide. The existing expertise in the relatively few diseases that are being targeted is limited, and intellectual interests will likely be diverted toward certain diseases, at least temporarily. Management oversight is equally limited, as the United States is faced with the dilemma of massive increases in demand on federal agencies to manage funds at a time when the general administrative and governmental trend is to downsize. This disjunction between supply and demand could potentially devastate the long-term capacity of the federal government to manage the response to intentionally or unintentionally introduced infectious diseases. The problem is compounded by the fact that great sums of money are being directed toward academic centers and other nongovernmental organizations, which could result in a brain drain from the federal sector and leave it at grave risk of managing the funds inappropriately. It is unclear how these problems should be addressed.

Despite the challenges and concerns outlined above, workshop participants suggested that if problems related specifically to the development of countermeasures for bioterrorism can be solved, the country will at least have begun to address some of the crucial issues related to the control and prevention of infectious diseases generally, such as access to medicines. It is hoped that over the next year there will be many such positive changes.

International Perception of Bioterrorism

It is crucial that issues related to biodefense spending be viewed in a context larger than the U.S. perspective on bioterrorism. In many countries, with the exception of some U.S.-owned establishments in foreign countries, bioterrorism is not perceived as a threat. Even in continental Europe, where much discussion about bioterrorism has taken place since the anthrax attacks in the United States and where more than 4,000 anthrax attacks, all hoaxes, have occurred in Germany alone, the total level of biodefense spending is less than $10 million, nowhere near the billions of dollars being spent in the United States. This difference illustrates markedly distinct priorities. The same is true in other parts of the world. Peru, for example, does not consider smallpox to be a high public health priority and is not prepared to invest large sums of money in addressing the possibility of a smallpox epidemic.

The United States cannot expect to receive the international cooperation that is critical to successful biodefense from parts of the world already suffering the enormous daily burden of infectious disease unless it also addresses the more immediate infectious disease–related concerns of other countries. It is unrealistic to expect other parts of the world to care about a handful of deaths from anthrax in the United States when they are experiencing such tremendous death tolls from TB, malaria, AIDS, and other infectious diseases. When developing biodefense programs and policy, the United States must integrate its own strategic needs with the real needs of its international partners.

On the other hand, although bioterrorism may not be a high-priority issue for every country, it would be in each country's best interest to improve its surveillance and laboratory capacity for the detection of infectious diseases in general, whether intentionally introduced or naturally occurring. Thus even if a smallpox outbreak or other bioterrorist act were never to occur, these countries would not be wasting their efforts. Moreover, as the number of anthrax hoaxes in Germany attests, such acts make demands on laboratory capacity. In Trinidad, for example, the Caribbean Epidemiology Center in Port of Spain responded to 20 requests for laboratory analysis of packages sent through the mail during the anthrax attacks in the United States; none of the packages was positive, and some even contained no white powder.

The Question of the Smallpox Vaccine Stockpile

Participants noted that international management of the smallpox vaccine stockpile is an important policy question that must be resolved. The United States is spending a large amount of money on the acquisition of smallpox vaccine, and other countries want to know whether they will have access to those supplies should the need arise. To many people in the developing world, much of the U.S. effort is considered self-serving. In the view of one workshop participant, not only is it untenable that a dose will be made available for every U.S. citizen, but the United States has no clear policy on intervening should smallpox occur elsewhere in the world. CDC has repeatedly said that any outbreak of smallpox anywhere in the world would be a global emergency requiring a U.S. response, but there needs to be greater clarity regarding exactly what this response would entail.

Scientific Freedom and Privacy Issues

Participants expressed concern regarding the impact of biodefense on scientific freedom. In particular, preventing the proliferation of biological weapons entails controlling technologies that may have multiple uses and may put scientific freedom at risk. How can the United States develop a nonproliferation regimen that provides security while also supporting scientific openness?

Privacy is also becoming a more serious issue as individual genome sequencing technologies become more sophisticated. Although information about personal genomes may be necessary for prophylaxis or treatment in the event of a bioterrorist attack, the use of such information raises questions about ownership and fair use.

EFFECTS OF THE DISSOLUTION OF THE FORMER SOVIET UNION ON PUBLIC HEALTH IN RUSSIA[8]

The post–cold war situation in Russia illustrates the public health impact of rapid socioeconomic change induced by globalizing forces in a country where state social programs were previously the sole provider of

---

[8]This section is based on the workshop presentations by Demin (2002) and Netesov (2002).

health and social safety nets. The dissolution of the Soviet Union in 1991 and the shift away from a bipolar world had public health repercussions not only in Russia, but also in Eastern Europe and worldwide. Although the situation in Russia is unique, it reflects what is happening globally in both the developed and the developing worlds: funding for public health and the public health infrastructure are failing, the health of migrants has become a key issue, and something must be done.

In the mid-1960s, the Soviet Union's public health and social security systems were comparable to those of many western countries. Until 1992, industry, the economy, and state social programs were all fueled largely by state exports of national resources, not manufacturing, and the labor population was of only secondary importance. Nevertheless, under the old Soviet "social contract," the social security of Soviet citizens was more comprehensive than was the case in most developed welfare states. When Russia began the process of liberalization in the early 1990s, however, the country was experiencing the peak of a major political and socioeconomic crisis. The hasty and unreasoned opening of the country to globalization processes during that difficult time has been identified as a key causal factor in the current public health crisis. The implementation of so-called "shock therapy" wiped out savings. The abolition of the state monopoly on foreign trade, natural resources, and alcohol turnover, as well as biased privatization of state property, created a small, deindustrialized economy oriented toward the export of raw materials that was beneficial for only a small segment of the population. The bulk of the population was deprived of economic power and was thus considered "excessive" during this early stage of post-Soviet reform (Demin, 2002).

The state abrogated its role in social security policy, the ruling elite overlooked the need for new approaches to social security, and privatization and the new market economy failed to substitute for the old Soviet state safety net. In 2002, about 30 percent of the population was living below the minimal standard. The total number of people living under conditions of poverty increased from 2.2 million in 1993–1995 to 57.8 million in 1997–1998. Fully 10 percent of impoverished individuals have reached a social low point and are rejected by society. At least one million children are neglected and homeless.

Russia is a geoeconomic vacuum, with a GDP only about 1.5 percent of the world average. Its external debt totals $138 billion, and about 25 percent of the state budget is earmarked to serve this debt. Considerable internal debt also remains. The outflow of capital in 2001 was an estimated $17 billion, which is comparable to the $15.9 billion foreign investment in Russia for the entire period between 1992 and 1998.

Since 1991, negative global influences—illegal drugs; self-destructive behaviors; and the marketing of tobacco, alcohol, and junk food products by transnational corporations—have intensified. Transnational tobacco companies control about 65 percent of local tobacco production, and the level of production of tobacco products in Russia increased from 150 billion cigarettes in 1990 to 400 billion in 2001. The country has experienced a parallel increase in the number of individuals who smoke.

Russia's current public health problems developed in parallel with but lagged behind its social and economic changes, as illustrated by the decline in public health following the economic crisis of August 17, 1998, which resulted in a fourfold devaluation of the national currency during a 2-week period. Many public health indicators have been steadily declining since 1964, despite two short periods of improvement from 1985 to 1987 and 1995 to 1998. Impoverishment has resulted in large-scale undernourishment and increasing rates of morbidity and mortality, and a considerable portion of the Russian population has become party to the vicious cycle of poverty, disease, and premature death. Infectious diseases are becoming more prevalent as living and social standards fall; the leading cause of death from infectious and parasitic diseases is TB, which killed about 30,000 people in 2000 (see below for additional statistics on rates of mortality from infectious diseases). In 2000, the average life expectancy in Russia was 59 years for men and 72.2 years for women. Lower life expectancy is particularly drastic among males as a result of poverty, substance abuse, and disease.

Russia's public health problems are further complicated by the reality that, because of insufficient funding, infectious diseases among the considerable flow of migrants from states of the former Soviet Union are neither monitored nor controlled. At present, Russia has about 5.5–12 million illegal migrants. By 2010, the number of illegal migrants in Russia is predicted to be as high as 19 million, representing 15 percent of the population. The situation is complicated by the fact that most of these migrants come from developing countries with unfavorable sanitary conditions, including Afghanistan and Iraq.

The administration of Vladimir Putin has developed revised policies for legal migration into Russia, along with revised pronatalist, health-promoting policies, in an effort to compensate for the current low rate of population growth. The death rate currently exceeds the birth rate by a factor of 1.7. As President Putin claimed in his first address to the national parliament on July 8, 2000, this rate of population growth is insufficient for the normal functioning of Russia, and if it continues will threaten the survival of the nation. President Putin predicted that the national population may decrease by as much as 22 million over the course of the next 15 years. In addition to the increase in the mortality rate, since 1990 some 100,000 individuals have left the country each year to obtain permanent residence abroad.

Russia's experience shows how even the availability of natural resources and an educated population cannot guarantee a country's integration into the global economy, nor can it ensure internal social stability or good public health if social security and public health are not identified as priorities as part of planned political, social, and economic changes. The ruling elite's underestimation of the importance of public health can have profound repercussions for national security; the economy; and survival at the national, regional, and global levels.

In 2001, the leading cause of death in the Russian Federation was cardiovascular disease (865.2 deaths per 100,000 persons), which is typical of most developed countries. The second was injuries, including homicides, suicides, accidents, and poisoning (225.2 deaths per 100,000); the third was cancer (203.9 deaths per 100,000); the fourth was pulmonary disease, including influenza, pneumonia, TB, and various other infectious and non-infectious diseases (65.1 deaths per 100,000); and the fifth was other infectious and parasitic diseases (24.3 deaths per 100,000). The sections below provide some specific infectious disease statistics, including, for comparative purposes, differences in rates of morbidity and mortality from hepatitis between Russia and the United States.

Hepatitis A[9]

From 1967 to 2001, morbidity and mortality from hepatitis A was much higher in Russia than in the United States. Although the figures from before 1990 are questionable because diagnosis was based mainly on etiology (the enzyme-linked immunosorbent assay [ELISA] test was not used for diagnosis until after 1990), the mortality rate in Russia has still been much greater than that in the United States. In 1967 there were approximately 1,500 deaths from hepatitis A per 100,000 persons in Russia, compared with fewer than 50 deaths per 100,000 in the United States. In 1990 there were slightly more than 1,500 deaths per 100,000 in Russia, versus nearly zero deaths per 100,000 in the United States. In the late 1990s, mortality rates in Russia dropped to fewer than 50 deaths per 100,000. Although the cause of this decline is unclear, it may have been due to a declining birth rate and a decrease in the population of children under 10 years of age. Nevertheless, a significant percentage of the population had no antibodies against the hepatitis A virus, and the mortality rate from the disease is again on the rise, approaching 100 deaths per 100,000 in 2001 (tempered in some outbreak areas by vaccination).

---

[9]This section is based on the workshop presentation by Netesov (2002).

Hepatitis B[10]

The situation with hepatitis B is similar to that with hepatitis A, with significantly greater mortality occurring in Russia than in the United States over the course of the past 25 years or so. In 1993, hepatitis B was responsible for between 150 and 200 deaths per 100,000 persons in Russia; by 2000, this number had risen to greater than 400. However, a significant decrease in morbidity occurred in Russia in the early 1990s, when the new, sensitive diagnostic ELISA test was introduced, resulting in quicker access to treatment. Unfortunately, the sudden drop was interrupted by a huge increase in intravenous drug use (a primary means of contracting the infection), which continues to this day (although there was a small decrease in 2003 due to the U.S. presence in Afghanistan, where the poppy fields are located).

Measles, Mumps, and Diphtheria

In 1993, there was a large increase in measles incidence in Russia, from fewer than 2,000 infections per 100,000 persons in 1992 to more than 4,000 infections per 100,000 in 1993. Although the jump in incidence was due in part to a vaccine shortage, it was caused largely by media propaganda and a widespread suspicion that the measles vaccination was harmful. Since then, however, the incidence of measles has fallen to practically zero.

A similar phenomenon occurred with mumps in Russia in the late 1990s, although there is still a significant incidence of the disease, despite the implementation of revaccination procedures. In 1995, there were fewer than 3,000 mumps infections per 100,000 people; this figure rose to almost 10,000 by 1999. By 2001, the incidence had dropped to fewer than 2,000 infections per 100,000.

Diphtheria incidence also experienced a dramatic jump in the mid-1990s, again because of both suspicion that the vaccine was harmful and a vaccine shortage. In 1992, there were fewer than 500 infections per 100,000 persons; in 1994, there were more than 2,000. The incidence is now less than it has been in over a decade and is continuing to decline.

Tuberculosis

Roughly 2 million people die each year from TB worldwide (WHO, 2002b), with the vast majority of these deaths (98 percent) occurring in

---

[10]This section is based on the workshop presentation by Netesov (2002).

developing countries (Mukadi et al., 2001). In 2000, approximately 8.7 million new TB cases were reported worldwide, of which an estimated three to four percent were multidrug-resistant (Jaramillo, 2002). In most countries, the average incidence of TB has recently been increasing by approximately three percent per year; however, the increase is much higher in Eastern Europe (eight percent per year) and African countries most affected by HIV (10 percent per year). Just 23 countries account for 80 percent of all new TB cases. In 2000, over half of these cases were concentrated in five countries: India, China, Indonesia, Nigeria, and Bangladesh. Although Zimbabwe and Cambodia report fewer total cases, they possess the highest global rates per 100,000 population (562 and 560, respectively) (WHO, 2001b). If present trends continue, more than 10 million new cases of TB are expected to occur worldwide in 2005, mainly in Africa and Southeast Asia; by 2020, nearly one billion people will be newly infected, 200 million will develop the disease, and 35 million will die (WHO, 2002a).

The global resurgence of TB is not confined to developing countries. From 1990 to 1995, TB incidence in Russia increased by 70 percent, with more than 25,000 persons dying from the disease each year (Netesov and Conrad, 2001). The increased incidence is compounded by the spread of multidrug-resistant TB, especially in prisons, where patients typically self-administer treatment. Because most prison clinics experience massive shortages of drugs, the majority of patients are unable to complete their full course of treatment, a situation that fosters the emergence of multidrug-resistant TB. Indeed, the rate of multidrug-resistant TB among TB isolates in Russian prisons is an astonishing 40 percent, compared with just 6 percent in the general population. The overall rate of TB per capita in prison populations (i.e., including both multidrug-resistant TB and other forms of the disease) is nearly 100 times higher than in the Russian population at large.

Syphilis

The estimated global burden of new cases of infection with *Treponema pallidum* among adults in 1999 was 12 million (WHO, 2001a). As with other sexually transmitted diseases, the greatest number of cases occurs in South and Southeast Asia and sub-Saharan Africa (four million each), followed by Latin America and the Caribbean (three million). Although the primary and secondary syphilis rates in the United States declined by 90 percent from 1990 to 2000, the disease remains an important problem in the South and among certain subgroups. The newly independent states of the former Soviet Union have recently seen a dramatic rise in syphilis rates, from 5–15 per 100,000 in 1990 to 120–170 per 100,000 in 1996 (WHO, 2001a).

HIV/AIDS

In less than 20 years, HIV/AIDS has become a pandemic requiring an unprecedented global response. More than 60 million people have been infected with HIV worldwide, and 20 million have died from AIDS, leaving an estimated 40 million adults and children living with HIV. Roughly 14 million children are living without one or both parents who died from the disease. In 2001 alone, it is estimated that five million people became HIV positive worldwide, 800,000 of them children (UNAIDS, 2002). Nearly one-third of those living with HIV/AIDS—11.8 million—are between 15 and 24 years of age (UNAIDS, 2002). Over the last decade, HIV/AIDS has increased dramatically in Russia. Although most people still contract the infection through intravenous drug use, more and more women are becoming infected through sexual transmission. As more women become infected, mother-to-child transmission also increases, causing a spillover into the general population. Specific projections of the number of anticipated HIV/AIDS cases are difficult because the incidence of HIV infection is declining in some populations and increasing in others, HIV testing continues to be voluntary, and reporting may be incomplete. Generally, the number of cases is expected to rise in areas where poverty, poor health systems, poor access to health care services, and gender inequality are prevalent; where resources for health care and prevention are limited; and where a high degree of stigma and denial is associated with HIV infection (Monitoring the AIDS Pandemic Network, 2000).

THE EXPERIENCE OF THE EUROPEAN COMMUNITY[11]

Many would agree that the development of the new European Community over the past 20 or 30 years has largely been a success story in both political and economic terms. Currently, the European Union comprises 15 states, and the hope is that it will expand eastward and add five new countries by 2004. Along with the success of the European Union, however, have come several new challenges associated with the movement of people, capital, and resources, all of which have important implications for the emergence, reemergence, and control of infectious diseases. The effects of

---

[11]This section is based on the workshop presentation by Kurth (2002). The Robert Koch Institute, a German federal institute, performs many of the same tasks carried out by the National Institute of Allergy and Infectious Diseases and CDC in the United States. The Institute conducts basic and applied research and is responsible for surveillance and other aspects of health reporting in both Germany and the European community in general.

this increased movement on infectious diseases and the manner in which the European Union responds could serve as a model for what might happen or could be done globally in the prevention and control of emerging infectious diseases. That being said, however, the accomplishments of the European community have arguably been more feasible than what will likely be the case in other regions of the world because European countries share common historical, cultural, economic, and religious backgrounds. At the same time, it is important to note that Europe has never intended to create a "United States of Europe." Rather, the intent is to remain a loose union of states, respecting the different nations' individual profiles and cultural differences.

Movement of People

There have been, and will continue to be, large movements of people across the borders within the European Union, as passports were abolished about four years ago. Within the Union, one can settle anywhere and attempt to make a living wherever one chooses. The labor market is free, and people are entitled to a job in any of the Union's 15 countries. This movement of people creates problems for the border countries, especially those to the south—Italy, Spain, and to a lesser extent Greece—where migrants and refugees from Africa and the Middle East first arrive. At present, as many have seen in the media, boats of refugees are turned back weekly, even though it is usually difficult to recognize where they have come from. Much of this movement is for economic reasons, and the problem is expected only to become worse in the future.

Not only is Europe the host of a large immigrant population, but Europeans, and especially Germans, also travel a great deal. Europeans make eight million trips overseas each year, involving 28 million border crossings. Thus, even though Europe is far north of the tropics, many tropical infectious disease killers, such as malaria, yellow fever, dengue, and even hemorrhagic fevers, are being imported on a large scale. In response to this situation, the European Union has established a Europe-wide rapid alert system, which is integrated into a larger worldwide rapid alert network.

Movement of Resources

The European community has probably been sharing resources on a much greater scale than could ever be achieved at the international level. Much of the current budget of the European Commission, which far exceeds $100 billion annually, is spent on infrastructural aid (e.g., establishing new factories and other activities and processes necessary to raise living standards). Before unification, Europe was divided into two economic regions: the poor (e.g., Portugal, southern Spain, Greece, and Ireland) and the rich (especially the areas surrounding Paris, Munich, London, and the Scandinavian countries). Unification has leveled these disparate living standards to some extent; today there is a smaller difference between the poorest and richest regions of Europe compared with poor and rich countries worldwide as described by workshop participants.

However, these same infrastructural efforts have also been associated with some negative developments. For example, an attempt was made to lower the cost of agricultural products by subsidizing them to an extent that was unfair to both the United States and developing countries, which generally have very little to sell to Europe except food.

Limits to Unification

The harmonization and standardization that characterize the unification of Europe have not proceeded without the deleterious influence of national egos. In October 2001, for example, when the consequences of September 11, 2001, were being discussed, there was talk about stockpiling smallpox vaccine. The discussion was terminated after only about 2 hours, however, when it became clear that no European country was prepared to have the stockpile stored or located in a different country. This unwillingness was due to apprehension that, should a crisis arise, the country with the stockpile would not deliver it as quickly as possible or as needed and agreed upon. The final decision was that each country had to have its own stockpile. Thus there are limits to globalization, even on the European scale.

REFERENCES

Acheson D. 2002 (April 16). *Globalization of the Food Supply.* Presentation at the Institute of Medicine Workshop on the Impact of Globalization on Infectious Disease Emergence and Control: Exploring the Consequences and Opportunities, Washington, D.C. Institute of Medicine Forum on Emerging Infections.

Barry M. 2002 (April 16). *Considering the Resources and Capacity for the Response.* Presentation at the Institute of Medicine Workshop on the Impact of Globalization on Infectious Disease Emergence and Control: Exploring the Consequences and Opportunities, Washington, D.C. Institute of Medicine Forum on Emerging Infections.

Cash R. 2002 (April 16). *Impediments to Global Surveillance and Open Reporting of Infectious Diseases.* Presentation at the Institute of Medicine Workshop on the Impact of Globalization on Infectious Disease Emergence and Control: Exploring the Consequences and Opportunities, Washington, D.C. Institute of Medicine Forum on Emerging Infections.

Cetron M. 2002 (April 16). *The World and Its Moving Parts*. Presentation at the Institute of Medicine Workshop on the Impact of Globalization on Infectious Disease Emergence and Control: Exploring the Consequences and Opportunities, Washington, D.C. Institute of Medicine Forum on Emerging Infections.

Corber S. 2002 (April 16). *A Response to the Shifting Trends*. Presentation at the Institute of Medicine Workshop on the Impact of Globalization on Infectious Disease Emergence and Control: Exploring the Consequences and Opportunities, Washington, D.C. Institute of Medicine Forum on Emerging Infections.

Demin A. 2002 (April 16). *Social Aspects of Public Health Challenges in a Period of Globalization: The Case of Russia*. Presentation at the Institute of Medicine Workshop on the Impact of Globalization on Infectious Disease Emergence and Control: Exploring the Consequences and Opportunities, Washington, D.C. Institute of Medicine Forum on Emerging Infections.

Freedman DO, Kozarsky PE, Weld LH, Cetron MS. 1999. GeoSentinel: The global emerging infections sentinel network of the International Society of Travel Medicine. *J Travel Med* 6(2):94–98.

Gardner P. 2002 (April 17). *New Directions in Capacity Building*. Presentation at the Institute of Medicine Workshop on the Impact of Globalization on Infectious Disease Emergence and Control: Exploring the Consequences and Opportunities, Washington, D.C. Institute of Medicine Forum on Emerging Infections.

Gordon D. 2002 (April 16). *The Global Infectious Disease Threat*. Presentation at the Institute of Medicine Workshop on the Impact of Globalization on Infectious Disease Emergence and Control: Exploring the Consequences and Opportunities, Washington, D.C. Institute of Medicine Forum on Emerging Infections.

Grondin D. 2002 (April 16). *Global Migration and Infectious Diseases*. Presentation at the Institute of Medicine Workshop on the Impact of Globalization on Infectious Disease Emergence and Control: Exploring the Consequences and Opportunities, Washington, D.C. Institute of Medicine Forum on Emerging Infections.

Heyman D. 2002 (April 16). *Invited Discussion: Response to the Shifting Trends*. Presentation at the Institute of Medicine Workshop on the Impact of Globalization on Infectious Disease Emergence and Control: Exploring the Consequences and Opportunities, Washington, D.C. Institute of Medicine Forum on Emerging Infections.

IOM (Institute of Medicine). 2000. *Ending Neglect: The Elimination of Tuberculosis in the United States*. Washington, D.C.: National Academy Press.

Jaramillo E. 2002. *DOTS-Plus & the Green Light Committee*. Presentation at "Meet the Expert" Session of the 33rd IUATLD World Conference on Lung Health, Montreal, Canada. Palais de Congres. WHO/CDS/STB/TBS. October 6–10.

Kimball AM. 2002 (April 16). *Considering the Resources and Capacity for the Response*. Presentation at the Institute of Medicine Workshop on the Impact of Globalization on Infectious Disease Emergence and Control: Exploring the Consequences and Opportunities, Washington, D.C. Institute of Medicine Forum on Emerging Infections.

Kurth R. 2002 (April 17). *The Global Application of Tools, Technology, and Knowledge to Counter the Consequences of Infectious Diseases: A Discussion of Priorities and Options*. Presentation at the Institute of Medicine Workshop on the Impact of Globalization on Infectious Disease Emergence and Control: Exploring the Consequences and Opportunities, Washington, D.C. Institute of Medicine Forum on Emerging Infections.

Leaning J. 2002 (April 16). *Health, Human Rights, and Humanitarian Assistance: The Medical and Public Health Response to Crisis and Disasters*. Presentation at the Institute of Medicine Workshop on the Impact of Globalization on Infectious Disease Emergence and Control: Exploring the Consequences and Opportunities, Washington, D.C. Institute of Medicine Forum on Emerging Infections.

LeDuc J. 2002 (April 17). *The Global Application of Tools, Technology, and Knowledge to Counter the Consequences of Infectious Diseases: A Discussion of Priorities and Options*. Presentation at the Institute of Medicine Workshop on the Impact of Globalization on Infectious Disease Emergence and Control: Exploring the Consequences and Opportunities, Washington, D.C. Institute of Medicine Forum on Emerging Infections.

Miller J. 2002 (April 16). *A Response to the Shifting Trends*. Presentation at the Institute of Medicine Workshop on the Impact of Globalization on Infectious Disease Emergence and Control: Exploring the Consequences and Opportunities, Washington, D.C. Institute of Medicine Forum on Emerging Infections.

Monitoring the AIDS Pandemic Network. 2000 (July 9–14). *The Status and Trends of the HIV/AIDS Epidemic in the World Symposium of the XIII International AIDS Conference*. Washington, D.C.: Monitoring the AIDS Pandemic Network.

Mukadi YD, Maher D, Harries A. 2001 (Jan 26). Tuberculosis case fatality rates in high HIV prevalence populations in sub-Saharan Africa. *AIDS* 15(2):143–152.

Netesov SV. 2002 (April 17). *The Current Situation and Perspectives of International Collaboration in the Field of Biomedical Sciences: The Example of the State Research Center of Virology and Biotechnology, VECTOR*. Presentation at the Institute of Medicine Workshop on the Impact of Globalization on Infectious Disease Emergence and Control: Exploring the Consequences and Opportunities, Washington, D.C. Institute of Medicine Forum on Emerging Infections.

Netesov SV, Conrad JL. 2001. Emerging infectious diseases in Russia, 1990–1999. *Emerg Infect Dis* 7(1):1–5. Erratum in: *Emerg Infect Dis* 7(3):491.

NIC (National Intelligence Council). 2000 (December). *Global Trends 2015: A Dialogue About the Future with Nongovernment Experts*. Washington, D.C.: CIA.

UNAIDS (Joint United Nations Programme on HIV/AIDS). 2002. *AIDS Epidemic Update*. UNAIDS/02.46E. Geneva, Switzerland: WHO.

UNAIDS and WHO. 2001. *AIDS Epidemic Update: December 2001*. UNAIDS/01.74E-WHO/CDS/NCS/2001.2. Geneva, Switzerland: UNAIDS/WHO.

Weis SE, Moonan PK, Pogoda JM, Turk L, King B, Freeman-Thompson S, Burgess G. 2001. Tuberculosis in the foreign-born population of Tarrant County, Texas by immigration status. *Am J Respir Crit Care Med* 164(6):953–957.

WHO (World Health Organization). 2001a. *Global Prevalence and Incidence of Selected Curable Sexually Transmitted Infections, Overview and Estimates*. Geneva, Switzerland: WHO.

WHO. 2001b. *World Health Report 2001: Global Tuberculosis Control*. Geneva, Switzerland: WHO.

WHO. 2002a. *Coordinates 2002—Charting Progress against AIDS, TB, and Malaria*. [Online]. Available: http://www.who.int/infectious-disease-news/ [accessed July 27, 2005].

WHO. 2002b. *Tuberculosis*. [Online]. Available: http://www.who.int/mediacentre/factsheets/who104/en/index.html [accessed July 27, 2005].

3

The Global Application of Knowledge, Tools, and Technology: Opportunities and Obstacles

C hanges in travel and trade and the disruption of economic and cultural norms have accelerated and made it much more difficult to control the emergence and spread of infectious diseases, as described in Chapters 1 and 2 of this report. Even as progress is made, the public health community will likely encounter further setbacks, such as growing antimicrobial resistance. Yet there is a positive side to these developments as well. While globalization intensifies the threat of infectious disease, it also results in stronger tools for addressing that threat. From technological advances in information dissemination (e.g., the Internet) to the growing number of bidirectional infectious disease training programs that are bringing clinicians, scientists, and students from both sides of the equator together, the opportunities made available by globalization appear as endless as the challenges are daunting.

At the same time, the opportunities afforded by globalization do not necessarily come easily. Workshop participants identified obstacles that, if not addressed, may prevent or retard the ability to take full advantage of some of these new global tools. Global surveillance capabilities made possible by advances in information and communications technologies, for example, are still fraught with numerous challenges. This chapter summarizes the workshop presentations and discussions pertaining to some of these opportunities and obstacles.

One of the most enthusiastically discussed opportunities made available by our increasingly interconnected world is the type of transnational public health research, training, and education program exemplified by the Peru-based Gorgas Course in Clinical Tropical Medicine. This program not only benefits its northern participants, but also helps build a sustainable public health capacity in the developing world. Historically, the goal of many tropical disease training programs was to strengthen the northern country's capacity for tropical disease diagnosis and treatment. The trend toward a bidirectional, more egalitarian approach that benefits the developing-country partner as much as its northern collaborator reflects a growing awareness that a sustainable global public health capacity can be achieved only with the full and equal participation of the developing world. Thus, not only are the Gorgas Course and other, similar programs becoming more popular, both politically and among students, but their nature is also changing in significant and telling ways. The shifting focus of many of the international training programs of the Fogarty International Center (FIC) within the National Institutes of Health (NIH) further reflects the increased awareness, funding, and efforts needed to strengthen bidirectional international training in epidemiology, public health, and tropical medicine in particular.

Are there enough of these programs to go around, however? In addition, despite the clear and growing need and interest, are U.S. medical and veterinary students receiving enough training in public health, let alone in tropical infectious diseases? The Gorgas Course, FIC programs, and other, similar initiatives are summarized here. The chapter also addresses the need to better incorporate public health training into U.S. medical and veterinary school curricula and ways in which Russian scientists could contribute to a transnational public health education program.

Workshop participants identified other opportunities for progress as well. These include worldwide access to antiretroviral agents and vaccines; an increased capacity for global and regional surveillance; and technological advances in information and communications technology, namely, the Internet.

Rather than focusing on specific opportunities, several of the presentations and discussions revolved around the various ways in which certain organizations and regions are capitalizing on such opportunities. The Pan American Health Organization (PAHO), for example, is relying on the development of regional political networks to aid in the construction of regional surveillance networks and to facilitate the sharing of diagnostic and treatment techniques across borders. Despite these promising developments, many obstacles impeding regional efforts to strengthen infectious disease control capacity remain.

Another regional example is Russia, which, despite its current general state of public health as described in the previous chapter, has experienced some recent achievements and taken advantage of opportunities for the development of international collaborations in infectious disease control. The State Research Center of Virology and Biotechnology (VECTOR) plays a leading role in these efforts, which are summarized here.

A final example is the relationship between the Massachusetts state public health laboratory system and public health clinics in Peru, whereby sputum specimens and isolates from Peru are sent to Massachusetts on a daily basis for drug resistance testing. This arrangement could serve as a model for a much larger, market-based approach to sharing limited public health resources.

TRANSNATIONAL PUBLIC HEALTH TRAINING PARTNERSHIPS[1]

As noted above, the trend toward bidirectionality in transnational education and training, whereby southern partners have as much to gain as their northern collaborators, reflects a growing awareness that a sustainable global capacity to respond to infectious disease threats requires the full and equal participation of developing countries where infectious diseases are endemic. It is vitally important that the intellectual, technological, and health care workforce capacities of the developing world be strengthened, both for the sake of improving the health of local populations and because so many of the world's infectious diseases arise in tropical countries and spread via nonindigenous travelers. One-third of all new infectious diseases identified over the past 25 years were discovered in Latin America. The Gorgas Course in Clinical Tropical Medicine and other international training programs offered by the Instituto de Medicina Tropical "Alexander von Humboldt" (IMT) in Lima, Peru, and several of the overseas training programs sponsored by FIC exemplify this trend toward bidirectionality, as described in this section.

Nevertheless, in addition to improving the capacity of the developing world, one of the primary goals of these programs remains the education and training of northern students, researchers, and practitioners. Despite the progress made over the past decade in providing increasing numbers of opportunities for U.S. students and health care practitioners to gain experience overseas, including experience with the treatment and control of tropical infectious diseases, much work remains to be done. Efforts of the American Society of Tropical Medicine and Hygiene (ASTMH) and others to improve the training of U.S. students in tropical infectious disease medicine are also summarized here.

Workshop participants expressed serious concern that too few medical and veterinary school students receive adequate public health training in general, let alone training in tropical infectious diseases. It is vital for front-

---

[1]This section is based on the workshop presentations by Barry (2002), Demin (2002), and Gardner (2002).

line practitioners to receive such training. As one participant observed, it was an astute physician who identified inhalational anthrax in Florida in the fall of 2001. This section includes a summary of the discussion pertaining to the need for public health training and the challenges, mainly monetary, that make meeting this need difficult.

Although most of the discussion of transnational training partnerships focused on collaborations between the developing and developed worlds, particularly between the United States and Latin America, participants also discussed how a global approach to public health education and training would benefit Russia, especially in light of rapidly developing antiglobalist and xenophobic sentiment in that country. Some examples of ways in which Russia could, in turn, contribute to a mutual exchange of information and skills were also outlined.

The Gorgas Course and Other Recent Bidirectional Training Initiatives: A Peruvian Perspective

Although U.S. and Latin American scientists have been collaborating for more than two decades, the collaborations have tended to involve only certain U.S. universities interacting with certain Latin American countries. This same colonial attitude has been true of European–African collaborations as well. The situation is changing, however. Developed-world partners are adopting new approaches in their interactions with the developing world and realizing that respecting the decisions made by their developing-country partners is critical to the long-term sustainability of these partnerships.

For example, IMT, on the campus of the Universidad Peruana Cayetano Heredia in Lima, where the Gorgas Course in Clinical Tropical Medicine is held, maintains a strong collaboration with the Belgian-run Institute of Tropical Medicine in Antwerp. An important component of this four-year collaboration is the way in which the Belgian partners have respected IMT's decisions. When the collaboration was initiated, the Belgians asked, "What is *your* priority? How would you like your Institute to develop?" A workshop ensued, IMT devised a plan, and the Belgians agreed with and supported the plan.

Another, more popular example is Peru's interaction with the University of Alabama (UAB) in support of the Gorgas Course in Clinical Tropical Medicine. This annual nine-week diploma course provides 380 contact hours (in English) and daily bedside teaching. Over the last six years, the Gorgas Course has trained 185 medical doctors from 44 countries. About 50 percent of the participants are from the United States, 17 percent from Canada, 12 percent from Latin America, 10 percent from Europe, six percent from Asia, five percent from Australia and New Zealand, and two percent from Africa. Most of the trainees are midcareer professionals with about 10 to 15 years of experience. Participants range from United Nations Children's Fund (UNICEF) project officers to missionary physicians, U.N. peacekeeping forces, and vaccine developers (see Figure 3-1). The age range of the participants is from under 30 to over 60.

The Gorgas Course does more than train. In two months alone there were some 10,000 visitors to cases published on its website. And since the anthrax attacks in the United States, there have been 7,000 U.S. inquiries regarding the anthrax photos provided by the Gorgas Course case collection. IMT also sponsors several other training programs and courses for professionals and students. For example, small grants are available for U.S. students to go to Peru for three or four months at a time and conduct research; two U.S. students participate each year and together have coauthored six published papers to date.

The bidirectional nature of IMT's relationship with UAB is illustrated by the approximately 20 Peruvian students who have trained at UAB over the last three years. In 2002 there were eight Peruvian residents in the UAB Department of Medicine, and the chief resident was from Peru. IMT also offers its own master's degree in infectious disease control, although this program is not yet as well supported as others. In recognition of the fact that IMT provides sustainable, credible training and is expected to continue to grow, UAB is undertaking several other new initiatives. In 2003, for example, IMT initiated a separate program for trainees from other Latin American countries, including Bolivia, Paraguay, Ecuador, and Colombia. UAB is also developing a plan to provide clinical training in HIV/AIDS and tuberculosis (TB).

Other Peruvian collaborations with the United States include a ten-year partnership with the University of Washington School of Public Health and Community Medicine; some 40 published papers have resulted from this collaboration. Several personnel from the University of Washington have also trained in Peru. Other examples include collaborations with the University of Maryland (cholera and typhoid fever), Johns Hopkins University (cysticercosis), and Harvard-affiliated Partners in Health (TB and multidrug-resistant TB).

In addition to respecting the decisions made by participants from the developing world, the adequate transfer of economic support is vital to the continued success of these types of programs. The failure to transfer sufficient funds to developing countries is one of the key issues regarding international partnerships. This is especially true of partnerships with the United States, as about 90 percent of U.S. funds designated for training programs in Latin American developing countries are actually spent in U.S. institutions. This is the case even when the award recipients are Latin Americans. In reality, the amount of funds transferred is very small, as the award money still belongs to U.S. institutions and private companies. The situa-

Post-Gorgas Course Activities I

Country	Activity
Albania, Angola, Congo, Kosovo, Liberia, Macedonia, Sudan	Mèdecins Sans Frontières assignments
Australia	Aboriginal Health Service
Bangladesh	UNICEF Project Officer
Bolivia (La Paz)	Medical Director, Food for the Hungry International
Brazil (Rio de Preto)	Teaching medical students
Cambodia (Phnom Penh)	Teaching psychiatry
Cameroon	Career missionary
Canada, United States	Opened travel medicine clinic (multiple graduates)
Chile, Germany	Opened first academic travel medicine clinic
Colombia (Medellin)	Leishmaniasis control program
Congo (Kinshasa)	Missionary physician
Cuba (La Habana)	Epidemiologist, Instituto Pedro Kouri
East Timor	NGO physician
Eritrea	UN peacekeeping with Canadian Armed Forces
Ethiopia	Established rural health clinic
Ghana	Career missionary
India (Pune)	HIV research

Post-Gorgas Course Activities II

Country	Activity
Iran (Tehran)	Teaching oral surgery
Kenya (Nairobi)	Head of Slovak mission
Latvia (Riga)	Head, Infectious Diseases Epidemiology Unit
Peru (Iquitos)	Malaria research, US Naval Medical Research Center
Peru (Iquitos)	STD research, UAB
Russia (Moscow)	University Teaching Faculty
Seychelles	Head, Communicable Disease Control Unit, MOH
South Africa (Capetown)	Pediatric TB fellowship
Thailand (Bangkok)	HIV clinical trials physician
Thailand	Vaccine development, Aventis Pasteur
Uganda (Kampala)	Teaching anesthesia officers
United Arab Emirates	Emergency medicine consultant
United States (Atlanta)	CDC EIS Officer, International Disaster Relief
United States (Bethesda)	NIH Malaria Vaccine Development Unit
Uruguay (Montevideo)	National Bacterial Resistance Program
Venezuela (Caracas)	Infectious Disease Faculty
Operation "Enduring Freedom" (location unknown)	Activated by US Special Operations Command

FIGURE 3-1   Post–Gorgas course activities I and II.
SOURCE: Barry (2002).

tion is analogous to American travelers who visit Peru but fly American Airlines, stay at the Sheraton or Marriott, and travel with a U.S. tour group. Although the trip may cost the tourist $3,000, only about $20 stays in Peru; the rest goes back to the United States (Gotuzzo, 2002).

The transfer of technology, skills, and knowledge gained from research endeavors in the developing world is another key issue. With regard to the transfer of technology, for example, the BACTEC system for drug suscepti-bility testing of *Mycobacterium tuberculosis* is available but cannot be used in Peru. With regard to the transfer of knowledge, it is critical that research conducted in developing countries have a significant, positive local impact. Even though European and U.S. countries have spent $1 billion on malaria research in just one African country over the past 50 years, the rates of mortality and morbidity from the disease have not changed, and the quality of life has not improved. This situation must be changed.

The Changing Nature of Fogarty International Center's Transnational Training Partnerships

The 35-year-old FIC has a specific mandate to promote and support international scientific research and training in the global health sci-ences and reduce global health disparities. In its early years, the agency focused largely on the exchange of scientists among developed coun-tries. Over the last 15 years, however, it has increasingly emphasized scientific capacity building and training in developing countries by awarding traditional training grants, mainly to universities within the United States. This shifting programmatic emphasis reflects the chang-ing nature of training partnerships between developed and developing countries. In addition, FIC maintains several mathematical modeling research programs addressing a wide range of issues, from disease preva-lence to rates of global mortality from influenza and the biomedical modeling of bioterrorism.

FIC's traditional training grants for capacity building and training have been highly successful. Foreign trainees come to the United States, where they receive clinical, laboratory, and research training in public health and then return to their countries, where they use their new skills in leadership oles. As a measure of FIC's success, one-quarter of the scientific presenta-ns at the World AIDS Congress in Durbin, South Africa, in 2000 had one more authors who had been trained with FIC support. In fact, these city-building programs have been so successful that they have reached int at which the foreign sites are now able to assume much more ibility and autonomy.

use of this success, FIC, in collaboration with its 10 NIH partners enters for Disease Control and Prevention (CDC), has established a new, next-generation grants program known as the International Clinical, Operational, and Health Services Research Training Award for AIDS and Tuberculosis (ICOHRTA-AIDS/TB). There are several important differences between this new approach to training individuals from overseas and the earlier, more traditional grants:

- Training site—Most significant is that, although the grants still fund collaborations, or partnerships, between sites in the United States and abroad, they are increasingly centered in the low-resource country. In the past, foreign trainees were brought to the United States, where they enrolled in courses and, in some cases, degree programs. Now, the training sites are increasingly located in the developing countries, and the developing-country participants set the agenda, decide whom to work with, and assume much more ownership of their efforts than in the past. This shift in emphasis empowers resource-limited countries to sustain their own health care initiatives without continued reliance on CDC and other outside agencies.
- Research agenda—In the past, research agendas were set mainly by grant recipients in the United States. The agendas of ICOHRTA-AIDS/TB will increasingly be set by individuals in the developing countries.
- Faculty mentoring—Faculty mentoring was previously performed mainly by faculty in the developed country. It is now being done increasingly by faculty in the developing country.
- NIH funding—In the past, NIH funding went to the site in the developed country. NIH funding now goes to sites in both the developing and developed countries; paired grants will include direct funding, including overhead costs, to both countries.
- Types of awards—The long-term sustainability of the grants program at a foreign site requires a long-term commitment from the United States. Traditional training grants are typically for five years, but these new-generation grants will be 10-year (or longer) cooperative agreement programs.
- Research emphasis—The earlier grants program focused mainly on epidemiology and prevention, important work without which these new-generation grants would not be possible. One of the primary goals of the new program, however, is to expand this focus and integrate clinical, operational, and health services research in an effort to apply results obtained at the benchtop to the bedside. The emphasis is on the integration of therapy and care with prevention efforts.

In addition to FIC's training grants programs, NIH oversees several other, similar international efforts, including the Prevention Trials Network, the Vaccine Trials Network, the Comprehensive International Program of Research on AIDS, Popular Opinion Leaders, International Centers for Excellence in Research, and Partnerships for HIV/AIDS Research in Africa. FIC also helps foster many major U.S. government and other international AIDS research efforts, including those of CDC's Global AIDS Program; the U.S Agency for International Development's Rapid Response Initiative; the Bill and Melinda Gates Foundation; the American Foundation for AIDS Research; the Elizabeth Glaser Pediatric AIDS Foundation; the Academic Alliance for AIDS Care and Prevention in Africa; and the Global AIDS, Tuberculosis, and Malaria Fund.

One of the most recently established FIC programs is the Global Health Research Initiative Program for New Foreign Investigators, a reentry grant program with the aim of reversing the "brain drain" from foreign countries that occurs when scientists come to the United States for graduate school and NIH training and do not return home. The program provides five years of support at $50,000 a year to scientists who reenter their home country after receiving training in the United States.

Also relevant is the International Training and Research Program in Emerging Infectious Diseases, a traditional program carried out at university sites conducting research overseas. In addition, FIC has partnered with the National Science Foundation and created the Ecology of Infectious Disease program. The purpose of this program is to support efforts toward understanding the ecological and biological mechanisms that govern the relationships between human-induced environmental changes and the emergence and transmission of infectious disease. Finally, FIC funds the International Studies on Health and Economic Development program, which supports projects examining the effects of health on microeconomic agents (individuals, households, and enterprises) and aggregate growth, as well as the effects of health finance and delivery systems on health outcomes.

Russia's Potential Contributions to Transnational Training

Although most of the discussion of international bidirectional training programs during the workshop focused on north–south collaborations, and U.S.–Latin American partnerships in particular, some participants commented on the need for a transnational public health research and education agenda in Russia, especially with regard to infectious disease control in migrant populations. Many Russian experts are capable of participating in such international collaborative programs, and Russia could contribute to this type of program in many ways:

• Russia's unique experience with protecting its population from extremely dangerous infections as part of the former Soviet Union's so-called "counterplot service" could be a very useful source of information for other countries.

- Russia could play a leading role in prevention and control programs for HIV/AIDS and other infectious diseases throughout Eastern Europe.
- Russia's stored smallpox specimens—one of the world's two supplies of wild virus—could be used for international collaborative research.
- Russian experts who are developing a register of sites in Russia where anthrax (*Bacillus anthracis*) spores are stored could contribute to an international effort to register and monitor anthrax sites around the world. Such a registry could be used in bioterrorism prevention and control, for example, to differentiate between bioterrorist and natural outbreaks.
- Russian experts could also aid in the development of a register of infectious disease carriers for use in preventing the dissemination of infectious diseases beyond national borders as a result of migration.

Recent Overseas Training Initiatives: A U.S. Perspective

After the Institute of Medicine (IOM) announced in a 1987 report, *U.S. Capacity to Address Tropical Infectious Disease Problems,* that only 300 people in the United States had the capability to diagnose and treat tropical diseases, ASTMH formed a committee to formulate recommendations for remedying the situation (IOM, 1987).[2] It was clear that the United States had no truly excellent program offering the kind of diploma training course, including laboratory and overseas experiences, called for by the IOM report. The ASTMH committee recommended that an examination in clinical tropic medicine be administered and that a diploma in tropical medicine and hygiene be offered. ASTMH distributed a request for proposal to 370 U.S. and Canadian medical schools; 22 schools responded, and the proposals from seven U.S. and five overseas medical schools were accepted. Today, there are strict requirements for a diploma course and a separate two-month overseas course. Since 1995, 619 individuals have taken the examination, 412 have passed, and 387 have had the overseas experience.

The Gorgas Course, which prepares students for the ASTMH examination, is an excellent example of the type of training program in tropical medicine and hygiene envisioned by ASTMH. In addition to the Gorgas Course, other ASTMH-accredited diploma courses are offered at the following universities: Bernard Nocht Institute (Germany), Case Western Re-

---

[2]ASTMH, a 1951 merger between the American Society of Tropical Medicine (formed in 1903) and the National Malaria Society (1940), is a major U.S.-based organization dedicated to the advancement of the study of tropical diseases and international health. Its goals are to promote and stimulate science-based policy in international health, professional interest and career development, and basic and operational research in tropical diseases.

serve University, Humboldt University (Germany), Johns Hopkins University, Liverpool School of Tropical Medicine, London School of Hygiene and Tropical Medicine, Mahidol University (Thailand), Tulane University, University of Virginia, West Virginia University, and Uniformed Services University of the Health Sciences.

A number of other ASTMH training initiatives were inspired by the 1987 IOM report. These include the Ben H. Kean Traveling Fellowships in Tropical Medicine (for clinical or research experiences for medical students and residents); the Centennial Fellowship (for senior undergraduate and graduate students to work on immunomolecular parasitology with colleagues in the developing world); the Burroughs-Wellcome Fund Fellowship (for overseas projects at collaborating field sites); the Gorgas Memorial Research Award (for Latin American and Caribbean scientists to work with their North American colleagues on collaborative projects); and travel awards for overseas colleagues to present their research at ASTMH annual meetings.

Many non-ASTMH educational initiatives have also emerged recently worldwide. They include the Yale World Fellows Program and the Yale/Johnson & Johnson Physician Scholars Program. The former attempts to bring together midcareer professional leaders from academia, government, nongovernmental organizations, business, and media from throughout the world in an effort to create an international dialogue and network among fellows and broaden the general understanding of globalization. Participants receive a generous stipend for themselves and their families so they can attend Yale for a semester or a full year. Fellows participate in seminars and independent studies during an initial visit; they revisit the campus after having worked back at their home sites for two years.

The Yale/Johnson & Johnson Physician Scholars program, which started in 1981, sends physicians-in-training in a variety of subspecialties to 16 sites around the world for overseas rotations. In 2002, when the program was broadened to include a national competition, it funded 65 scholars, including senior midcareer physicians. The goal is to place physicians in underserved areas where they can learn to recognize tropical diseases and develop long-standing bilateral relationships between their home school or hospital and the host area.

Not only there is a need for more training in tropical infectious diseases among health care providers in the United States and other countries in the developed world, but there is also a strong student demand for such training. By going abroad, students learn about and encounter diseases and conditions, such as measles, that do not occur regularly or at all in the United States. In 1984, just four percent of graduating medical students participated in overseas training. This percentage has risen dramatically. According to an unpublished 2002 study of nearly 400 internal medicine residency programs, 45 percent of those programs offered overseas training electives; another 45 percent expressed interest in developing such electives.

Students who have spent time abroad usually return to their home institution full of excitement about international and other career possibilities that they might otherwise not have considered. According to one study, physicians who participate in the Yale School of Medicine's International Health Program are much more likely, as they pursue their careers, to care for patients who require public assistance, immigrants, HIV-positive patients, and substance abusers (Gupta et al., 1999). The results of that study, however, are obviously affected by a selection bias, as not all physicians-in-training choose to undertake such overseas electives.

Despite the successes of the various overseas training programs described above (e.g., the Gorgas Course and FIC's overseas programs) and the need and student demand for more of these opportunities, many ongoing programs have several problems that need to be addressed:

• Participants often do not receive a sufficient preparatory curricular and cultural introduction to their programs and host sites.
• Trainees often lack the ability to speak the language of the host site.
• The programs lack a standardized curriculum across schools.
• Training places a potential burden on host sites. As the demand for overseas training and the number of students involved increase, this burden will become greater.
• The demand for overseas training opportunities is very high, but the supply of good mentorships is very low.
• There is a lack of bidirectional support—for example, funding to bring overseas faculty back to the United States for minisabbaticals.

Content of Medical and Veterinary School Public Health Curricula

The concern that most medical and veterinary school students are not receiving enough general public health education, let alone training in tropical infectious diseases, was discussed above. Most medical school curricula still offer only an hour or less of instruction in antibiotic resistance and the mechanisms of action of antibiotics. As noted earlier, some physicians practicing today have never seen a case of measles, and some veterinarians practicing today have never encountered foot-and-mouth disease.

Although training in tropical infectious diseases should constitute a significant component of the public health education of medical and veterinary school students, it is important to keep in mind that not all infectious disease problems emerge in the developing world. The United States is experiencing many problems within its own borders that need to be addressed. For example, the Alabama state health commissioner indicated at a recent public health forum on emerging infections that not enough diphtheria-pertussis-tetanus vaccine boosters are available to be administered to the next generation of Alabamians, and several audience members at that forum said they had taken their children to receive tetanus shots only to be told that there was no tetanus vaccine available.

A workshop participant noted that as a result of the 2001 anthrax attacks and the increased threat of bioterrorism, both real and perceived, instructors are generally spending more time on the pathogenesis and treatment of infectious diseases, particularly those that would result from the release of potential bioterrorist agents, and that the American Medical Association has been working on additions to the curriculum. However, the general perception is that the curriculum is already full, and in fact, the Liaison Committee on Medical Education has indicated that students today have too much contact time and need fewer lectures and more hours of small-group learning sessions.

Another participant suggested that perhaps medical and veterinary school curricula could be modified to incorporate public health training programs—both general programs and those focused on tropical infectious diseases—without necessarily increasing contact time. However, the cost of doing so could be prohibitive. U.S. academic centers are currently under great financial stress because of the obligations placed on them as a result of requirements promulgated at both the state and national levels. Most of this financial stress is a consequence of state balanced budget amendments and continuing reductions in levels of reimbursement by federal payers, despite inflationary pressures. This situation is occurring in the face of growing numbers of uninsured and indigent patients, who are disproportionately and largely cared for by academic health centers. Moreover, fewer physician-scientists in the United States are applying for NIH grants and conducting research than in the past, and the number of M.D.'s applying for grants is declining in proportion to the number of applying Ph.D.'s. The recently increased NIH budget and the new influx of funding for biodefense (see the discussions of funding in Chapters 2 and 4) will certainly help alleviate this situation to some extent, but they are not solutions. It is worrisome that medical research institutions may be too preoccupied with other matters to take full advantage of the unprecedented opportunity offered by the new biodefense funding.

Thus, although the participants generally agreed that medical schools have an obligation to teach physicians about global public health and to equip them with cultural competence within the realm of health care, they also acknowledged the severe financial pressures that currently plague academic health centers. These financial pressures, which are expected to worsen in the future, combined with an already full curriculum, make curriculum modification a difficult challenge.

Finally, a participant suggested that training and research consortia and collaborations among U.S. academic institutions be established to make better use of limited funding and resources. This has already been accomplished to a limited extent but could be done much more effectively. The key may lie with NIH, CDC, or other funding programs with the power to promote these kinds of collaborations. One goal of such collaborative programs would be to take advantage of the expertise that exists in different places so as to avoid duplicated or fragmented efforts. The focus would be on one or two collaborative sites and on doing what needs to be done to make those sites truly excel, rather than on dividing the funding among multiple sites.

REGIONAL EFFORTS TO TAKE ADVANTAGE OF GLOBAL OPPORTUNITIES[3]

Three regional or organizational efforts have been undertaken to take advantage of some of the newly available global tools and opportunities: (1) PAHO's efforts to prevent the spread of infectious diseases in the Americas; (2) Russia's effort to build new international bridges in the wake of post-Soviet reform; and (3) a partnership between the Massachusetts state public health laboratories and Peruvian health clinics that serves as a model for a novel, market-based approach to sharing limited public health resources. This section summarizes these efforts.

Regional Efforts in the Americas: Global Opportunities and Obstacles

The original mandate of the 100-year-old PAHO was to help countries work together to prevent the spread of communicable diseases. While having broadened over time, the original mandate remains fundamental. Communicable diseases are still a major public health problem throughout the Americas, as recent outbreaks of emerging and reemerging infectious diseases in the region attest. PAHO's 1995 Regional Plan to Control Emerging and Reemerging Diseases identified four major steps necessary to address this continuing threat. Other organizations, such as the World Health Organization (WHO) and CDC, have identified the same steps as priority needs worldwide:

- Improve surveillance.
- Strengthen the public health infrastructure through laboratory capacity building and training.

---

[3]This section is based on the workshop presentations by Cash (2002), Demin (2002), Miller (2002), Netesov (2002), and Timperi (2002).

- Improve the means used to translate the findings from applied research into simple diagnosis and treatment techniques, including methods that can be used in the field.
- Develop a capacity for outbreak detection, primarily by formulating prevention and control guidelines or manuals and conducting training programs.

PAHO's efforts to take these steps illustrate how some of the new opportunities made available by globalization are being or can be used on a regional scale. For example, improved information and communications technologies allow faster cross-border communication. PAHO is currently assisting Central American countries with the development of INFOCAM, an electronic system that will allow routine sharing of surveillance information. Also being used are e-mail, electronic chat rooms, and the Program for Monitoring Infectious Diseases (ProMED)—an Internet-based reporting system dedicated to rapid and global dissemination of information on outbreaks of infectious diseases that affect human health. Despite these many opportunities and early success stories, however, much remains to be done.

Opportunities

Several political networks have developed throughout the region, and these, in turn, have encouraged more cross-border cooperative efforts to prevent and control the emergence and spread of infectious diseases. Examples include the following:

- Caribbean Community (CARICOM), RESSCAD (meeting of the health sector of Central America), Mercosur in the southern cone of South America, and Hipolito Unanue in the Andes comprise countries that have joined together not only to improve their economic situations, but also to enhance infectious disease surveillance efforts and develop regional health plans.
- Caribbean countries have developed a subregional plan for HIV/AIDS, which has been signed by all their health ministers. Such a collaborative effort is especially critical in this region, where migration among countries is an important factor in the transmission of HIV.
- With CDC support, countries have banded together and agreed on the priority syndromes they will strive to address. For example, the countries in the southern cone of South America have assigned priority to efforts against hemolytic-uremic syndrome and influenza, and the countries of the Amazon basin to efforts against sudden adult death, hemorrhagic fevers,

and malaria. The countries run certain laboratory tests to detect the agents responsible for these syndromes and then report their results. Extensive in-country training occurs to strengthen laboratory capacity and the capabilities of laboratory clinicians.

• Nineteen countries are participating in two networks that evaluate the antimicrobial resistance of several organisms.

• Nine countries in the Amazon basin have held regional meetings to address malaria-related issues.

• Three subregional laboratory surveillance networks have been established in the Americas: one in the Amazon basin, one in the southern cone, and one in Central America.

• A regional laboratory network for food analysis has been set up in the Americas, and all countries in the region are now using the Hazard Analysis Critical Control Point Inspection model for the inspection of food-processing establishments. Several regional meetings have been held to determine how the risk of bovine spongiform encephalopathy can be assessed and what steps must be taken to investigate any reports or suspicions.

• Southern cone countries have agreed to work together and meet annually to discuss efforts to control Chagas' disease. Their collective efforts have already reduced the spread of the disease vector (through the spraying of thatched houses with insecticide), and the seroprevalence of the disease among schoolchildren has decreased by 90 percent.

Regional political developments have made it easier to share various diagnostic and treatment techniques. This, coupled with increased, faster travel, has also made it easier for people from different countries to come together for training; for example, training in detecting and responding to outbreaks has occurred in all South American and several Central American countries. The sending of specimens to regional reference laboratories for analysis has been facilitated as well. Along with CDC in Atlanta, Georgia, several regional laboratories are now acting as reference laboratories as well as training centers.

Finally, because of globalization, free trade, and the critical role of participation in the world market in a country's economic development, countries throughout the Americas have generally become more motivated to improve their public health. For example, as was witnessed in the United Kingdom, the economic repercussions of foot-and-mouth disease can be devastating. The rapid control of the 2000–2001 South American outbreak of foot-and-mouth disease demonstrated not only the importance of communicating and working together, but also the economic benefits of doing so. The certification that Uruguay and Argentina were free of disease, for example, increased their exports to the United States by billions of dollars.

Obstacles

Despite the many successful regional efforts to strengthen the capacity to prevent and control the emergence and spread of infectious diseases in the Americas, numerous obstacles remain. These obstacles are not necessarily unique to PAHO or the Americas. In a sense, although globalizing forces have in many ways made countries working together to control the spread of local outbreaks more feasible, in other ways they have made it more difficult:

- As important as immediate intercountry communication is to the rapid detection and control of local outbreaks, many countries hesitate to report such outbreaks because they fear the potential economic repercussions. If a country were to announce that it was experiencing a dengue, cholera, or foot-and-mouth disease outbreak, for example, not only would tourism plummet, but so, too, would the country's exports. Most countries would prefer to try to control an outbreak without broadcasting its occurrence.

- It is important to note that the purpose of rapid intercountry communication is not just to prevent the spread of local outbreaks, but also to aid in the detection of local outbreaks that may already have spread. A generation ago, the epidemiology of food-poisoning outbreaks might have been limited to church picnics, where everybody got sick in the same place. Now, with so much international travel and the global transport of food, infectious disease cases arising from one source may appear in other locations very far away. Identifying cases of disease in disparate geographic locations that have arisen from the same source poses a great challenge.

- As the world becomes more international, there is a growing need to comply with international standards for the interregional and transcontinental movement of goods and products, such as standards imposed by the World Trade Organization (WTO). Many countries are being forced to improve previously ignored conditions in order to export goods. They are also being forced to develop credibility. When a country says it is free of a certain disease, has tested a certain product, or has carried out a certain inspection, people must be able to believe it.

- Sometimes, when a food product does not meet export standards, it is consumed or sold locally. Another major challenge has therefore become ensuring that food consumed or sold locally is of standard export quality, and that improvements countries are making in their production and food-processing practices are countrywide and not confined to their export industries or factories.

- Finally, to improve public health, it has become necessary to work outside regular health channels and target everyone at the community level, from vendors to street children and favelas.

After the workshop presentation on PAHO's regional efforts, a participant asked about PAHO's role in Cuba, a country that has the lowest rate of HIV infection in the Americas and that has done a reasonably good job of controlling dengue, and yet either is not recognized for its public health efforts or is being punished in other ways. In response, it was pointed out that PAHO is simply a forum for the exchange of ideas among countries and that U.S. policy toward Cuba is not a PAHO issue. Cuba does in fact take part in many of the same PAHO training sessions and joint meetings in which the United States participates.

Russia: Opportunities for International Partnerships in a Borderless World

A critical but little appreciated factor in the achievement of smallpox eradication was a remarkable collaboration between WHO, the USA, and the USSR beginning in 1966 and extending through the certification of eradication in 1980. Although many years during this period were especially tense ones in East-West relationships, professionals from two countries worked together . . . to bring the smallpox eradication campaign to a successful conclusion.
—Henderson, 1998, p. 113

Over the past decade, Russia has been witnessing the emergence and reemergence of multiple infectious diseases, from hepatitis B to HIV/AIDS. These crises, coupled with the fact that the percentage of research funding allocated to the life sciences is far less than that in most other developed countries, has put the country in a precarious public health situation. Yet as much as globalization and the breakdown of cold war borders and social structures may have contributed to this situation, they have also provided opportunities for the development of international collaboration in emerging infectious disease research and prevention.

VECTOR plays a leading role in Russia's participation in various international cooperative efforts to prevent and control the emergence and reemergence of infectious diseases, and serves as an excellent example of the type of international collaboration made possible in a borderless world. VECTOR is located in Koltsovo, in the Novosibirsk region, the geographic center of the Russian Federation. Novosibirsk is the third-largest city in the Russian Federation and is located about 1,000 kilometers from the border with Mongolia and China and about 400 kilometers from the border with Kazakhstan.

VECTOR is organized into three main divisions: Research, Production, and Support. The Research Division includes six research institutes (Research Institute of Molecular Biology; Research Institute of Aerobiology;

Research Institute of Bioengineering; Research, Design, and Technology Institute of Biologically Active Substances; Research Institute of Cell Cultures; and Research Institute: Collection of Cultures of Microorganisms), as well as the WHO Collaborating Center for Orthopoxvirus Diagnosis and Repository for Variola Virus Strains and DNA. The Production Division produces pharmaceuticals and provides energy, water, and heat. The Support Division includes an animal breeding and holding facility and service and transport departments.

The center is involved in multiple public health research and disease prevention endeavors encompassing a wide range of infectious agents, including a collection of about 120 smallpox virus strains that SCR VB Vector scientists are studying in close cooperation with the United States and WHO. Moreover, the center is the only civilian institution in Russia where researchers work with Ebola and Marburg viruses. Additional agents with which VECTOR works include other human and animal pathogenic orthopoxviruses, tickborne encephalomyelitis virus, Japanese encephalomyelitis virus, Crimean-Congo hemorrhagic fever virus, hemorrhagic fever virus with renal syndrome, hepatitis viruses (A, B, and C), cytomegalovirus, herpesviruses, measles and mumps viruses, Venezuelan equine encephalomyelitis virus, rubella virus, HIV types 1 and 2, influenza viruses, some endemic animal and fish viruses, and multidrug-resistant TB.

The center is producing two immunobiological products for public health. The first is an innovative hepatitis A vaccine (Hep A-in-Vac), a cultured, inactivated, injectable vaccine for use against viral hepatitis A in adults and children. Hep A-in-Vac is unique to Russia, where VECTOR has been producing it since 1997. Second is an injectable vaccine against measles. VECTOR is the second-largest producer of a vaccine against measles in Russia, after the Moscow Enterprise of Viral Preparations.

VECTOR has also developed a range of diagnostic test kits that are currently being produced in the Production Division, and in some cases by shareholder companies. Infections or agents for which kits have been developed include: HIV, hepatitis (A, B, C, and D), tickborne encephalitis, measles, cytomegalovirus, toxoplasmosis, lues (syphilis), chlamydiosis, herpes, rubella, toxocariasis, opisthorchiasis, trichinosis, and helminthiasis.

Funding for Life Sciences in Russia and the United States

Funding for life science research in the United States has increased almost constantly over the last four decades in terms of both the absolute amount and the relative percentage of all (except defense-related) science research funding. By 2000, funding for life science research had reached almost 50 percent of all nondefense science research funding. The situation in Russia is very different. According to the Russian Foundation of Basic Research (RFFI), the main source of competitive research funding in Russia, life science funding in 2001 represented less than 22 percent of all science research funding. Because RFFI does not fund defense science, these figures indicate that the relative percentage of life science funding in Russia is more than two times lower than that in the Untied States.

Unfortunately, the same is true of foreign and international funds awarded to Russian scientists. For example, in 2000 only 25 percent of all Cooperative Grants Program awards to Russia were in the biological sciences. In 1999, only 18.6 percent of all funding from the International Science and Technology Center (ISTC), the main funding source for science research in Russia, was for biotechnology and life sciences. The latter figure has risen during the past couple of years to about 24 percent, but it is still well below the 50 percent level in the United States. Over the past several years, the number of ISTC-funded VECTOR projects has increased from less than five in 1995 to 25 or 26 in 2002. In addition to ISTC, other international programs from which VECTOR receives funding include the Civilian Research and Development Foundation in the United States; the International Association (INTAS) of the European Community; the North Atlantic Treaty Organization science program; the Initiatives for Proliferation Prevention (IPP) Program of the U.S. Department of Energy; FIC; and the Volkswagen Foundation in Germany.

International Collaboration

Several recent achievements in public health in Russia can be attributed to the increasing collaboration between VECTOR and the various international funding agencies and programs cited above:

• One of the first ISTC grants helped VECTOR complete preclinical trials and organize clinical trials for its hepatitis A vaccine, which has been in production since 1998. Although VECTOR started developing the vaccine in the mid-1980s, a shortage of funds in the mid-1990s delayed its dissemination.

• VECTOR has been collaborating closely with several international and foreign agencies, including WHO, CDC, and the U.S. Army Medical Research Institute of Infectious Diseases (USAMRIID), on smallpox virus research. One of the first grants was from WHO in the early 1990s, with which VECTOR started sequencing smallpox virus genomes in cooperation with some Moscow-based institutions. The current collaboration (with CDC and USAMRIID) involves daily e-mail exchanges and sometimes direct television connections.

• International collaborations have allowed the rapid development of new and improved Enzyme-Linked Immunosorbent Assay (ELISA) diagnostic test kits for the detection of disease markers.

•   International collaborations have led to the sequencing of the genomes of many viruses endemic in Russia, including orthopoxviruses and current isolates of hantaviruses, viral hepatitis, and Congo-Crimean hemorrhagic fever virus. This sequencing information will be helpful in the development of new diagnostic kits and initiation of the development of recombinant vaccines.

•   VECTOR has participated in international efforts to develop methods for the rapid detection of multidrug-resistant TB. The Novosibirsk region has one of the largest prevalences of TB in the Russian Federation and a high percentage of multidrug-resistant TB.

•   VECTOR has participated in about 30 training courses on good manufacturing practices (GMP) and good labor practices (GLP) to improve the quality of production of pharmaceuticals, diagnostic kits, and vaccines.

•   Finally, VECTOR was the second Russian institution to register its ethical committee with NIH. This move has helped the center take an active role in introducing ethical principles and share its knowledge with medical clinics and other institutions in the region.

VECTOR has many current and proposed goals and activities, including:

•   Study of the prevalence and the properties of pathogens that represent either a natural or a potential bioterrorist threat to public health and animal husbandry in the Asian part of Russia and neighboring countries.

•   Continued laboratory and diagnostic support for the identification and localization of infectious disease outbreaks.

•   Continued development of a new generation of techniques for the diagnosis, prevention, and treatment of infectious diseases in both humans and animals, which could also be used in the event of a bioterrorist attack.

•   Continued participation in improving both national and international biosafety regulations and developing local epidemiological response plans.

•   Continued development of information technology–assisted means of predicting infectious disease outbreaks and identifying emerging human and animal pathogens.

•   Creation and operation of a research and educational complex for the improvement of professionally skilled experts in the fields of biosafety, epidemiology, GMP, GLP, and good control practices.

•   In the event that the proposed International Center in VECTOR is created, a long-term strategic collaboration that is far less subject to the political and economic fluctuations of member states.

The Need for a New Public Health Paradigm in Russia[4]

Despite the achievements of VECTOR and its participation in various international collaborative efforts, an enormous amount of work remains to be done in Russia with regard to strengthening public health capacity. Of the four sectors that will play key roles in shaping the next stage of post-Soviet public health reform—private enterprise, civil society, the state, and international players—the state must play the central role in breaking the vicious cycle of poverty, inequality, disease, premature death, and depopulation that currently plagues Russia. The capacity of private enterprise remains compromised in Russia, and civil society is still underdeveloped. International partnerships, such as those sustained by VECTOR, will be vital to the state's success.

To capitalize on the international partnership opportunities made available by globalization, however, it will be crucial to overcome the gap between the reality and the image of post-Soviet changes in Russia within both the Russian political and international arenas. Within the former arena, the Russian dialogue on globalization has been inadequate and has been centered on accession to WTO and globalization's impact on specific economic interests. The effect of globalization on health is not mentioned in many official documents, including those of the Russian Ministry of Health, or in a number of other important, recently released government documents. In the international arena, public health and globalization issues should be considered for inclusion in the activities of the Russian–U.S. intergovernmental commission on health, and major international organizations and foreign governments implementing programs in Russia must direct more attention toward the social and public health aspects of their proposed changes. Programs based on irrelevant standards and developed for other types of societies at different stages and levels of development are unsustainable in Russia and collapse when external support and funding are exhausted.

A participant noted that the Cooperative Threat Reduction program, the scientific cooperation between former Soviet scientists and their western counterparts that was established for the purpose of fighting infectious disease and sharing knowledge, is in considerable jeopardy at the moment. The Bush Administration can no longer certify that Russia is committed to honoring and abiding by the terms of the Biological Weapons Convention and, as a result, will no longer request money for new projects or additional spending on ongoing cooperation projects on which approximately $350

---

[4]See also Appendix D.

million has already been spent. This situation will continue until either the U.S. Congress provides the administration with a waiver of the certification requirement or Russia becomes more forthcoming about its previous activities during the Soviet era and permits greater transparency into its ongoing biological research programs. This is a very worrisome development.

A Public Health "Bank"

Because limited global public health resources must be used in a cost-effective and conservative manner, the only way the public health sector will be able to respond effectively to the increasing globalization of infectious disease is by pooling the resources of all participants. If this cannot be accomplished, individual countries, especially those in the developing world, will never be able to afford everything they need to manage increasingly globalized infectious diseases, nor will public health as an institution be able to protect its credibility. A workshop participant introduced as a possible solution establishing a public health "bank" to pool resources that could be shared across borders.

Although the majority of public health tasks are accomplished by the private sector and the amount of work done in the public sector is small by comparison, the public sector has a unique credibility. Public health is called upon when problems cannot be readily solved or when unexpected outbreaks overwhelm either short- or long-term capacities. Its credibility has been earned because the public health system has maintained timely, effective responses and good disease prevention policies and practices.

To sustain this credibility, however, public health needs a critical mass of resources, including sufficient technology, staff, and capital, to continue to provide effective services and products. Technology must keep pace with the rapid changes that continually occur, staff are needed to maintain expertise over time, and capital is required to sustain the services and products provided through economic ups and downs. It is virtually impossible to maintain this critical mass of resources on an individual statewide or even countrywide basis. Collaborative efforts may be the best if not the only solution.

In this light, a participant suggested that public health adopt a market-like architecture that would be operable on a global level and would allow the movement of resources across political barriers. The establishment of some type of public health "currency" would facilitate the sharing of resources and provide a conduit through which the developed and developing worlds could exchange experiences and information. When public health professionals learn how to manage problems in the developed world, where they have enormous resources at their disposal and are exposed to relatively few infectious diseases, it is difficult for them to attain the proficiency necessary to deal adequately with problems in the developing world, which has few resources and an enormous infectious disease burden.

Moreover, a market-like architecture would make use of the extensive capabilities and expertise of state public health laboratories, which today often are not being fully utilized. Members would contribute their assets to the bank and make them accessible on demand; a global health broker, such as WHO or some newly created organization, would manage the enterprise. A daily, ongoing, collaborative commitment would be necessary. For example, even though case rates of TB are minuscule in the United States, TB testing and intensive high-technology diagnostics are routine nationwide. This represents an enormous U.S. public health resource waiting to be used in a more meaningful way.

The relationship between the Massachusetts state public health laboratory and clinics throughout Peru can serve as a model for this market-like architecture. As noted earlier, the Massachusetts state public health laboratory receives on a daily basis sputum specimens and isolates that have been collected from Peruvian clinics for the detection of *Mycobacterium tuberculosis*, which causes TB. After the isolates in the samples have been tested for drug resistance, the results are reported back to practitioners in Peru, again on a daily basis. By using specimens from Peru that are much more difficult to assess than those to which they would otherwise be exposed, the Massachusetts laboratory workers are benefiting from a specific 4-week training program. Thus, the capacity of the Massachusetts laboratory is being developed while it is simultaneously providing real-time testing for drug-resistant TB in Peruvian patients. That the bank is mutually beneficial to all partners is an important selling point to political leaders (Timperi, 2002).

Other participants expressed interest in this notion of a global public health resource bank, even though it is unclear how the bank would operate. One participant suggested that a bank of this sort might be a useful construct for establishing bidirectional training programs in infectious disease control.

DRUG AND VACCINE ACCESS AND DELIVERY IN THE DEVELOPING WORLD[5]

Vaccines and antiretroviral agents have enormous proven public health benefits and could potentially save millions of lives in the developing world. Yet while globalization should be making it more feasible to bridge the gap in their access and delivery between the developed and

---

[5]This section is based on the workshop presentations by Miller (2002) and Redfield (2002).

developing worlds—for example, by increasing technology transfer—many obstacles remain.

Barriers to Implementing Vaccination Programs in the Developing World

Vaccine programs are one of the most successful tools for addressing public health concerns in an equitable manner. The history of global vaccination initiatives—particularly the Children's Vaccine Initiative (CVI) and the Global Alliance for Vaccines and Immunizations (GAVI)—suggests potential areas of improvement for the global public health system.

Before 1974 and the eradication of smallpox, routine vaccination for childhood diseases was implemented in less than 5 percent of the global birth cohort and in very few developing countries. An expanded immunization program, which initially included six antigens—those for diphtheria, pertussis, and tetanus; oral poliovirus; *Mycobacterium bovis* BCG (bacillus Calmette-Guérin), and measles—and subsequently yellow fever was launched in the mid-1970s.

A decade later, in 1985, the IOM report *Vaccine Supply and Innovation* (IOM, 1985) led to the rapid expansion of NIH research and the development of new vaccines by the U.S. military. In 1990, UNICEF introduced universal childhood immunization, which achieved about 80 percent coverage throughout the world. During the same year, those efforts led to the World Summit of Children and the launch of CVI, whose charge was to accelerate the development and deployment of vaccines globally.

The global history of vaccine usage over the past two decades, however, reveals a growing gap between developing and developed countries in the numbers of vaccines that have been introduced successfully (see Figure 3-2). Although countries have been encouraged during this time to recognize the value of immunization for infectious disease control, most countries have faced operational and financial constraints.

GAVI was formed in 2000 in response to this situation; its financial arm, the Global Vaccine Fund, was initially capitalized by the Bill and Melinda Gates Foundation with more than $750 million. This vaccine purchase fund was designed to serve the 78 poorest countries, that is, countries with a gross national product (GNP) under $1,000. Other barriers to implementing vaccines on a global basis besides per-dosage cost were not taken into account.

To help identify such barriers, a study on routine hepatitis B vaccination worldwide was conducted in the late 1990s. It was found that, despite a recommendation by WHO that all countries introduce universal vaccination against hepatitis B, in 1998 only about 75 of 179 countries or territories with populations of more than 150,000 were actually administering the vaccine. This is a vaccine that costs 50 cents per dose and prevents a

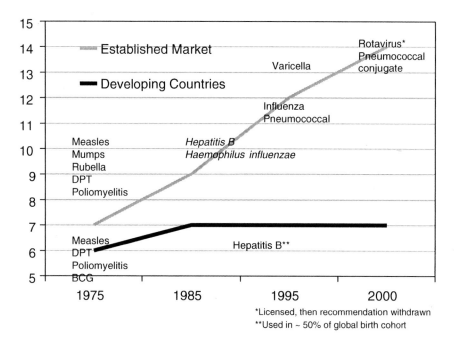

FIGURE 3-2 Number of vaccines used routinely in developing and developed countries.
SOURCE: Miller (2002).

bloodborne, sexually transmitted disease that leaves about 20 percent of those infected carriers for life. Yet it was not being used (Miller, 2002).

The study revealed that the two most important predictors of whether a country would adopt the hepatitis B vaccine were its coverage rates for other vaccines and the cost of the vaccine relative to per capita Gross Domestic Product (GDP). Also, countries that spent more money on treatment costs were five times as likely to adopt the vaccine, and those with a greater disease burden, as measured in years of life lost, were more likely to adopt than those with a lesser burden. When these factors were incorporated into a logistic regression model that was then applied to other vaccines, such as that for *Haemophilus influenzae* type B, the model achieved 87 percent accuracy in predicting which countries would be most likely to adopt new vaccines and in what order. It is interesting to note that these countries were not always those GAVI had targeted; that is, they did not necessarily have a per capita GNP below $1,000. Rather, with few exceptions, they were the countries with the worst infrastructures.

Since its inception, GAVI has recognized that infrastructure is an important, albeit complex, issue that must be addressed. How the needed infrastructure should be built, however, and what role GAVI can play must be determined. Numerous challenges exist, including the following:

- Translation or adaptation of new public health interventions—The implementation of any type of health intervention in a new setting must take local conditions into account.
- Technology transfer—Building infrastructure requires understanding the technical limitations of the setting and the need to use locally appropriate technologies. Recently, for example, large-scale campaigns have been carried out in response to outbreaks of meningitis that have ravaged the sub-Saharan African region; many of these campaigns have relied on 50-dose vials of vaccine with five syringes. One can imagine the number of iatrogenic transmissions of bloodborne pathogens that result from such a program.
- Political commitment—Building local infrastructure requires political commitment and a certain level of civil society and governance to oversee the effort. Often, even though United Nations (UN) countries' organizations and ministries of health are involved, there is no involvement at the national level. It may be necessary to approach the problem at a much lower level of government or society.
- Human resources—The ongoing lack of human resources and appreciation for local health interventions is another key constraint. To attain GAVI's goal of vaccination coverage rates in excess of 80 or 90 percent, there must be personnel on the ground. Although an epidemiologist can be parachuted in to meet critical, short-term needs, such an approach does not address long-term infrastructural needs and the sustainability of personnel at the local level.
- Economic barriers—The creation of the Global Fund to Fight AIDS, Tuberculosis, and Malaria (Global Fund) and the contributions of new global public health partners will help alleviate economic barriers to building infrastructure.
- Oversight—Some type of evaluation process that is not self-serving will be needed to achieve long-term accountability.
- Commitments of private suppliers—Vaccination programs rely on public–private partnerships and commitments from private suppliers, which in turn expect credible demands. As a result of the sudden ramp-up of GAVI, critical vaccines are in short supply. Without credible demands that are backed financially, serious problems will be encountered. For example, even though whole-cell pertussis vaccines are still being promoted in much of the developing world, soon no company may be manufacturing them.
- Absorptive capacity—In the rush to achieve desirable short-term outcomes, local programs tend to be scaled up through increased humani-

tarian assistance. The sudden introduction of billions of dollars into these systems, however, raises the question of how rapidly this money can really be spent wisely. Although these efforts may be well intentioned, they often exceed the absorptive capacity at the local level and lead to what is termed "programmatic iatrogenesis," in which the cure is worse than the problem (Miller, 2002). For example, although it was a noble goal, the introduction of a malaria eradication program promoted both vector and parasite resistance (when, for example, local farmers started using DDT for purposes other than malaria control). As another example, a lack of long-term planning, combined with a lack of local recognition of unsafe drug injection practices and the need for appropriate technology, has raised many issues regarding schistosomiasis control in Egypt. Finally, expanded vaccination efforts, including eradication programs, raise questions about whether vaccination should cease following eradication. Economically, it makes sense to push for eradication efforts. Once an agent has been eradicated, poor countries have no incentive to continue vaccinating. If the agent comes back in one or two generations, however, hundreds of millions of people around the world will be susceptible to the disease.

Several steps must be taken to address the above challenges:

- Governance—Many countries do not have a functional ministry of health or planning that can adequately oversee health programs. Therefore, other levels of government or even local academic institutions or nongovernmental organizations will need to take on this role.
- Appropriate policy for local needs—It is critical that policy be directed toward local needs. To this end, FIC intiated the Disease Control Priorities Project (DCPP) in response to a 1993 World Bank Development Report. Currently DCPP's partners include the World Bank, WHO, FIC, and the National Library of Medicine (NLM); they examine disease control priorities in terms of both intervention needs and science and technology capabilities.
- Economic barriers—Long-term planning and a long-term financial commitment based on science, not politics, are crucial. The new influx of global funds directed toward international public health is a step in the right direction (see Chapter 4). However, there is some question as to how long the Gates Foundation, for example, and other large foundations are going to remain committed to GAVI and other programs.
- Human resources—FIC recently undertook a study to demonstrate to WHO and its Commission on Macroeconomics and Health that human resource capacity is as much a global good as is product development. Indeed, product development in the absence of personnel at the local level who can use the product is only half the job. FIC has several programs in

place to address this issue. Most recently, for example, to reverse the brain drain, the Global Health Research Initiative Program for New Foreign Investigators has been providing grants for foreign nationals trained in the United States to return to their home countries (see the discussion earlier in this chapter). Ultimately, one of the greatest hopes for the future lies in training foreign nationals who then assume prominent positions within the governments of their own countries.

•   Appropriate technologies—The implementation of successful vaccine programs requires not only improvements to appropriate technologies, but also assurance that adequate funding for these technologies and a commitment to their proper use are directed specifically at resource-poor populations. Public–private partnerships are important to this end, but unless additional support and incentives are provided specifically for communities with few resources, this will be a difficult barrier to overcome. For example, although safer equipment for vaccine delivery may not be a priority in the United States, where safe injection practices are already in place, it may be critical for resource-poor populations.

•   Understanding of local incentives—Infectious diseases and infectious disease control can be understood only within the larger social science or anthropological context (see Chapter 4 for additional discussion of the social context of epidemiology). This context includes local incentives to implement vaccination programs.

Access to and Delivery of Antiretroviral Agents in the Developing World

Antiretroviral therapy is currently the only tool available for mitigating the economic and social destabilization due to HIV/AIDS in sub-Saharan Africa, a situation that may spread to India and other parts of the world. This is the case despite the tremendous resources that have been expended on development of an HIV vaccine. Despite its promise, however, the introduction of antiretroviral therapy into resource-limited settings poses many challenges. Of primary concern is the emergence of drug-resistant virus (IOM, 2005).

It is expected that over the course of the next 10 years, 30–50 million Africans will die from HIV/AIDS. Although poor health and death do not necessarily lead to political instability, they do maintain the economics of poverty. The continuously decreasing life expectancy in the region will progressively affect both the industrial workforce and the family unit, leading to the destabilization of society. As many who have worked in sub-Saharan Africa have witnessed, orphans are already raising orphans, and fathers have lost the ability to train their children in many agricultural skills. In the absence of intervention, this destabilization will worsen and, as noted, may spread to other regions.

From a foreign policy perspective on global health, antiretroviral therapy has several goals:

- To reduce the impact of the HIV/AIDS pandemic on declining life expectancies in the countries affected.
- To reverse the tragic trend of the increasing number of orphans whose parents have died from HIV-related causes.
- To reverse the trend of the loss of key members of the workforce, including local industrial workers and teachers.
- To minimize the impact of the pandemic on local governments and global economics.
- To avert the development of economic and political instability in sub-Saharan Africa and the spread of this instability to other regions of the world.

Lessons to Be Learned from Antiretroviral Use in the United States

The introduction of antiretroviral therapy in the United States has had a major, positive impact on mortality (death from advanced HIV infection) and morbidity (conditions secondary to HIV infection), but it has also raised many important issues. First, disparities in access to health care have made it more difficult to implement antiretroviral therapy effectively in the African American community, where a significant number of individuals are experiencing treatment failure as a result of drug resistance. Second, increased morbidity and mortality have occurred secondary to drug-induced toxicities. Third, the rate of transmission of drug-resistant virus has increased. Finally, there have been significant shifts in consensus recommendations on how antiretroviral therapy should be used. To further complicate matters, there are currently 18 antiretroviral drugs available, but they are not interchangeable; each has its own profile that makes it more or less suitable for use in resource-limited settings.

Both in the United States and in Europe, antiretroviral therapy has been associated with a high rate of treatment failure in the first year (e.g., 63 percent of the patients in a Baltimore clinic, 53 percent of the patients in a Cleveland clinic, 50 percent of the patients in San Francisco General Hospital, and 40 percent of the patients in an Amsterdam clinic). A key factor contributing to such high failure rates in the first year of therapy is impatience for progress and the premature introduction of new treatments into the HIV-infected population. Before antiretroviral agents were introduced into the United States in 1985, there existed a lack of significant public health debate regarding consensus recommendations for use of the drugs, a poor understanding of the goals of treatment for the prevention of HIV replication in vivo, and a lack of debate about the premature use of antiretroviral therapy and its effect on the future ability to control the epidemic. The wide-scale application of consensus treatment guidelines occurred before the effectiveness of several drug therapies—zidovudine [AZT] monotherapy, sequential monotherapy, and combination therapy with two nucleoside analogues and one protease inhibitor—had been validated by clinical data. For these therapies, particularly those involving protease inhibitors, the pharmacokinetics were pushed beyond their capacities. Furthermore, the lack of approval or preapproval of drugs as a result of the findings of drug–drug interaction studies resulted in significant alterations in pharmacokinetic interactions. This, in turn, led to the use of subtherapeutic doses and the development of drug resistance.

The requirement for strict adherence to the treatment regimen for these drugs has also contributed to viral resistance, an especially important point to keep in mind when the drugs are introduced into resource-limited settings. The drugs should be used in the context of directly observed therapy and in the presence of treatment helpers, mother's helpers, or treatment support systems. According to one study, even 95 percent adherence (e.g., one or fewer missed pills per week in a 21-pill-a-week regimen) can lead to a 20 percent failure rate (Paterson et al., 1999), while 90 percent adherence (missing two or fewer pills per week) can lead to a 50 percent failure rate.

Because of drug resistance, antiretroviral treatments have since their inception evolved from the initial AZT monotherapy to combination therapy to salvage therapy. Between 30 and 60 percent of all patients receiving treatment in the United States are infected with a drug-resistant HIV strain; approximately 10–15 percent of patients are infected with strains with cross-resistance to at least three classes of drugs and are on deep salvage therapy because their resistance to virtually all antiretroviral drugs leaves them no other treatment options; and about 14 percent of new infections are caused by drug-resistant virus. The negative repercussions of the premature introduction of antiretrovirals must be kept in mind when these drugs are made available in resource-limited areas.

In addition to drug resistance, other constraints on the use of combination antiretroviral therapy in resource-limited areas of the world include toxicity and side effects, drug–drug interactions, issues of adherence to and the complexities of the regimens, a lack of long-term efficacy in real-life settings, a loss of HIV-specific immunity, and cost. Thus there are real questions about the feasibility of antiretroviral therapy for most people in the world in need of treatment.

The Need for an African Solution

There is growing awareness, both within and outside of Africa, of the need for an African solution for HIV/AIDS. A number of African leaders are interested in the potential of antiretroviral therapy, largely because they are concerned about the survival of their democracies. The Group of Eight (G8) countries are also becoming more aware of the problem; the Global Fund, for example, was developed specifically to provide assistance for the treatment of AIDS, along with TB and malaria.

In fact, now that HIV/AIDS has become a national security and foreign policy issue for the developed world and the resources for intervention are no longer limited to traditional international health programs, this is an opportune time for the introduction of antiretroviral agents into Africa. Moreover, antiretroviral therapy has become more feasible from a clinical standpoint. Three or four very potent reverse transcriptase regimens with low pill burdens are available, as are some excellent drugs with good potencies that can be administered once a day, some with high mutation thresholds. Cost reduction efforts by the pharmaceutical industry and potential contributions from the Global Fund also enhance the feasibility of introducing the widespread use of antiretroviral therapy into Africa.

Although the development of an African solution involving the use of antiretroviral agents must proceed aggressively, the effort must also be undertaken with great caution. The current American approach of sequential combination chemotherapy and sequential drug failure is obviously not a durable formula for slowing or reversing the economic and social destabilization caused by HIV/AIDS in Africa. If viral resistance were to emerge in sub-Saharan Africa, no amount of economic or political will be able to control the epidemic. Thus the most critical aspect of an African antiretroviral solution is to take the necessary steps to prevent the emergence of drug-resistant virus. These steps include the following:

• A sustainable strategy for antiretroviral treatment in resource-limited settings needs to be developed, implemented, and evaluated; this strategy should be aggressive but prudent and should be different from the U.S. approach of sequential combination antiretroviral therapy. For example, one approach would be to evaluate the feasibility of alternative strategies for reducing mother-to-child transmission among pregnant and nursing women, and then expand feasible strategies to the greater adult population.

• There is an urgent need for debate on timing antiretroviral therapy so as to avoid the premature introduction of suboptimal therapy and the resultant emergence of drug-resistant virus. The best available knowledge needs to be applied to identify the optimum regimens for wide-scale use. A number of African countries have proudly provided zidovudine-lamivudine (Combivir) to their patient populations; however, this practice should be curtailed until a more effective strategy can be developed. Nigeria has decided to use stavudine, lamivudine, and nevirapine, but again, this may not be an optimal decision based on the drugs' mutation thresholds and current understanding of how the drugs work. At the very least, the effectiveness of the drugs should be demonstrated prior to their wide-scale use by a population. Only drugs that have excellent potency profiles, high mutation thresholds, and limited toxicity profiles and to which there is limited cross-class viral resistance should be used. Use of the currently available protease inhibitors is not feasible in resource-limited areas.

• In light of the above issues, the evaluation of alternative treatment strategies in resource-limited settings ought to be a scientific priority.

• Directly Observed Treatment-Short Course (DOTS) is perhaps the most critical element of any antiretroviral treatment strategy, at least initially. The mutation thresholds for individuals with viral loads greater than 50 copies of RNA per milliliter of blood plasma are much higher than those for individuals with viral loads below 50 copies per milliliter, and pilot studies have shown that DOTS can achieve 100 percent suppression rates. DOTS enhances adherence; prevents drug leakage from public pharmacies into the informal sector, which will likely be a significant problem in resource-limited areas; prevents the use of counterfeit drugs; maximizes the ability to recognize early drug toxicities; decreases the need to monitor patients for their viral loads and viral resistance, given that the 100 percent suppression capacity of the regimens has been validated; and provides a support system for individuals while teaching them the skills required to maintain successful therapy.

• Product profiles and selection criteria need to be developed for resource-limited areas. For example, one of the most important criteria as regards preventing the development of resistance is for the drugs to have high mutation thresholds.

• Attainment of generic status for selected products should be accelerated, if necessary.

• The development of new treatments designed for use in resource-limited settings needs to be prioritized.

• The primary care infrastructure in Africa needs to be strengthened.

• African health professions education and the local health professions workforce need to be improved.

• The political will to do what is necessary over the long run, including making the priority decisions required to prevent economic and political instability, needs to be developed.

• The operational capacity of the Global Fund needs to be enhanced.

Whatever action is taken in sub-Saharan Africa will have historic consequences; indeed, it will shape the world of the twenty-first century. If the approach used in sub-Saharan Africa is successful, it could be extended to other regions, with broad economic and political consequences around the world. If it is unsuccessful, the AIDS epidemic will continue to widen the health and economic gaps between the developed and developing worlds and exacerbate the growing political instability in Africa and beyond.

Antiretroviral Therapy as a Global Public Good

Some of the issues addressed during the discussion of antiretroviral therapy in Africa raised questions about drug development and drug delivery in general. Given the complexities and implications of the economics of the pharmaceutical and vaccine industries, it was suggested that an in-depth discussion of this important topic be reserved for a separate workshop or other venue involving economists, among others. Nonetheless, some participants made a few comments on the subject, which are summarized below.

The terrible inequities and disparities that characterize the HIV/AIDS crisis in Africa have led many people to argue that antiretroviral therapy should be considered a global public good, and that as such, the drugs should be provided free of charge to all who need them. There is concern, however, that identifying antiretroviral agents as a global public good would create a situation whereby pharmaceutical companies would begin undergoing the same adverse selection phenomenon currently being experienced by health insurance plans in the United States.[6] Public health interventions that are cost-effective for the public are not a source of profit for manufacturers. As people turned to companies that provided free antiretroviral products, the companies might consider those products a wasted investment and decide to abandon their production. At the workshop, this situation was compared to the pressure that has been exerted on vaccine companies to provide vaccines for only a few cents per dose. In the 1980s, there were about 20 vaccine manufacturers; today there are only four major manufacturers, and only two of these are in the United States. Neglecting to

---

[6]Adverse selection in health plans refers to the selection of less expensive (i.e., with lower premiums), suboptimal health insurance plans by low-risk consumers and the selection of more expensive (i.e., with higher premiums), higher-quality health plans by high-risk consumers (e.g., immunocompromised or elderly patients). Low-risk consumers choose plans with fewer benefits but lower premiums, so they are not subsidizing high-risk consumers. High-risk consumers are more likely to pay the higher premium for a better plan because there is a greater chance that they will actually need the care provided. Therefore, the sickest customers make up a smaller pool of higher premium–paying individuals, and eventually it becomes too expensive for health insurance companies to provide the necessary care to these higher-risk patients. Consequently, companies must raise their premiums even higher or eliminate the plans altogether. In a sense, as one participant said, high-quality plans that provide the best care are ultimately punished for doing such a good job.

consider the market conditions for vaccine products may drive even these few remaining vaccine manufacturers out of business.

The same situation applies to companies that sell products for both the prevention and treatment of the same disease. If it is more cost-effective, from a public health standpoint, to take preventive measures for a given disease, these companies will make more money by developing and producing preventive products and will have less incentive to develop and produce the corresponding treatment products.

Finally, it was noted that when these issues are discussed, people often start thinking immediately about the need for new drugs. However, the 23 percent rate of implementation of DOTS noted several times during the workshop illustrates that, at least in the case of multidrug-resistant TB, the main problem is not the production of new drugs but the implementation of the therapy. Even if the pharmaceutical industry produces a new anti-TB drug every year, multidrug-resistant TB is going to continue to emerge worldwide unless the implementation of DOTS is improved. As anti-HIV therapies are introduced into countries, it must be kept in mind that for many reasons, there may be fewer innovative efforts to develop new therapies in the future. The same is true of antibiotics. Thus it is crucial that the first steps taken be the right ones.

OPPORTUNITIES FOR AND OBSTACLES TO GLOBAL SURVEILLANCE[7]

Effective in-country surveillance systems are one of the many reasons smallpox was and remains eradicated.[8] As noted throughout this report, however, emerging infectious diseases are no longer geographically contained; therefore, effective in-country surveillance systems alone cannot prevent and control their global spread. A global surveillance system is necessary to better protect against infectious diseases through a collaborative response.

An effective global surveillance and response system has four key components: accurate surveillance, appropriate information dissemination, a

---

[7]This section is based on the workshop presentations by Cash (2002), Cleghorn (2002), Corber (2002), and LeDuc (2002).

[8]A number of additional factors contributed to the successful eradication campaign: the epidemiology of the disease was understood; the disease could be easily recognized; a low-cost, effective technology (i.e., the bifurcated needle and a vaccine) was available; there was a clear political commitment and an understanding that eradication had local and global benefits; and there was a willingness to help those countries that were too poor to conduct eradication efforts by themselves.

reasonable international response, and adequate enforcement by multilateral agencies. Ideally, clinical identification of an infectious disease in the field would be followed by diagnostic laboratory support, and finally diagnostic confirmation by a regional, national, or international laboratory, such as WHO, which would also establish an international strategy appropriate for the situation. The international response would involve WHO or another agency that would disseminate the information and coordinate the support. Nations would then institute their own control procedures on the basis of their national policies, international regulations, WTO policies, and, if necessary, Codex Alimentarius Commission food standards. Eventually, the outbreak would be controlled with minimal international spread and disruption of trade.

However, there are several impediments to the establishment of such a global surveillance and response system. Perhaps most important, regional and local health officials sometimes face strong political pressure to suppress outbreak reports so as to protect the country from the potentially damaging economic and political costs that often ensue. These costs stem in part from the lack of dissemination of information or the dissemination of inappropriate information by health officials and the media, as well as the limited diagnostic, treatment, and prevention capacities available in developing countries. The media are often prone to sensationalism when reporting on outbreaks. Other nations may issue travel advisories or impose trade sanctions, even when such measures are unnecessary, in an effort to protect their populations, public confidence, political interests, and industries. Indeed, the measures taken all too often are far more stringent than is necessary or appropriate.

The 1994 outbreak of plague in India serves as a disturbing example of what can happen when a country reports an outbreak. The outbreak, which caused 56–60 deaths, occurred in the town of Surat, which at the time was experiencing economic and environmental conditions among the worst in the country. India's diagnostic capacity was not very good at the time, and there was some question as to whether the outbreak actually involved plague. On the basis of its assessment that the outbreak was plague, however, India responded in accordance with WHO health regulations and ensured the adequate monitoring of both people and goods. Nonetheless, when the public was informed of the outbreak, many people fled from Surat, including physicians, who were among the first to leave (after treating suspected cases and instituting control measures such as the distribution of antibiotics). Although WHO recommended that there be no restrictions on trade and travel, trade restrictions were imposed by Qatar, the United Arab Emirates, Bangladesh, Oman, Italy, Sweden, and others. Moreover, Italy, France, Germany, Canada, the United Kingdom, the United States, and other countries restricted travel to India, and more than 2.2 million tourist trips to the country were canceled. Overall, the reported outbreak cost India an estimated $2.3 billion in lost trade and travel; the country experienced a record trade deficit in 1994.

Why was the response to India's reporting so extreme, given that its actions were appropriate according to the recommendations of WHO, and especially given that it was unclear whether the outbreak was in fact plague? Ironically, a small, confirmed outbreak of plague occurred in the western United States at the same time.

The cholera epidemic in Peru in 1991 serves as another example of the negative repercussions of outbreak reporting. The epidemic began on the Peruvian coast and then traveled south through the Amazon basin into Brazil (even though the reported mortality rate was less than one percent, which may have been due to underreporting). Peruvians made the diagnoses, informed the public, treated suspected cases, and instituted control measures. Signs indicating that people should treat their food and water to prevent cholera were posted throughout Peru and the rest of Latin America. Despite these measures, several of Peru's neighbors, including Bolivia, Ecuador, Chile, and Argentina, imposed trade restrictions (although the epidemic spread to Ecuador and Chile anyway). The European Union also imposed trade restrictions. Peru lost more than $700 million in trade, and Chile lost $330 million. Travel from North America and the European Union was restricted, and half of all tourists scheduled to travel to the region canceled their plans. These travel restrictions were instituted even though both CDC and WHO stated that "on no account should travel be restricted because of cholera." The United States implemented testing procedures and placed restrictions on imported food, despite the claim of the UN Food and Agriculture Organization that "there are no documented outbreaks of cholera resulting from commercially imported food. Epidemiological data suggest that the risk from contaminated imported food is negligible." The trade restrictions, lost tourism, and increased inspection that resulted from the reported cholera outbreak cost Peru more than $1.5 billion.

Other examples of the economic costs of outbreak reporting include the shift in coffee prices and subsequent trade-related economic losses that occurred as a result of the 1998 cholera outbreak in Ethiopia. Similarly, the 1998 Nipah virus outbreak in Malaysia, which led to trade and travel restrictions, as well as the loss of the local swine production–related infrastructure, cost the country hundreds of millions of dollars. The current situation with regard to tourism in the Caribbean is another good example of the tension between reporting an outbreak and withholding information to avert economic loss. Because tourism is such a significant industry in the Caribbean—more than 50 million people visit the region each year, many of whom arrive on massive cruise ships—the economic impact of outbreak reporting would likely be quite significant. For this and other reasons, much remains to be done to develop an effective regional surveillance system in the Caribbean.

Anecdotal evidence suggests that many countries suppress the reporting of information on outbreaks. Pakistan, for example, has experienced many cholera outbreaks over the past 35 years, none of which have been reported. HIV/AIDS is commonly underreported or not reported at all in many countries, while known plague outbreaks in Africa and elsewhere have gone unreported as well. This is not surprising, as there is no reason to expect that a farmer raising livestock in Argentina, for example, would let it be known that his cattle are dying from what appears to be bovine spongiform encephalopathy.

To encourage the rapid and accurate reporting of outbreaks and to strengthen global surveillance and response capacities, three main challenges must be met:

- The economic and political costs of outbreak reporting must be minimized:

    —Governments and trade associations must be better educated.

    —WTO and WHO need to be proactive in preventing inappropriate economic responses.

    —Economic aid should be granted to countries that are treated unfairly.

    —Mechanisms for the rapid redress of inappropriate responses need to be developed. Decision makers and policy makers need to be aware that if such a situation is not resolved quickly, individuals may lose their livelihoods through the loss of their perishable products.

- The dissemination of inaccurate information must be remedied:

    —Transmitting accurate information early in an outbreak is critical to a prompt and appropriate response. Press releases and other reporting information (e.g., from WHO, CDC, national health organizations, and nongovernmental organizations) need to be reliable and credible.

    —The media (television, print, and radio, as well as the Internet and the World Wide Web) need to be better educated with regard to their role in outbreak reporting, and it must be determined who is responsible (e.g., the government or schools of public health) for educating those who are doing the reporting. Reporters need to be educated in the principles of surveillance, the true threat of outbreaks, the importance of transmitting accurate information, and the impact of stigmatization and sensationalism. The last point is especially important: too often the victim is blamed, and too often the victim is a poor person in a poor country.

- The limited assistance available for diagnostic, treatment, and prevention capabilities must be rectified. The ability to diagnose, treat, and prevent outbreaks locally must be strengthened by improving the training of local field staff; strengthening national and local laboratory capacities; supporting research on inexpensive, easy-to-use detection methods and equipment; and increasing the transfer of existing biotechnology and genomics. For example, the Sustainable Sciences Institute in San Francisco, California, teaches investigators throughout Latin American about simple, inexpensive polymerase chain reaction techniques. Such programs need to be expanded and further supported, and the transfer of biotechnology and genomics needs to increase. Countries must be empowered to make diagnoses themselves rather than depending on CDC and others. Such dependency is not sustainable and does not give countries the capacity to deal with future outbreaks.

In addition to meeting the above challenges, workshop participants suggested a few other steps that could be taken to improve global surveillance. For example, clinical microbiology laboratories, which lie at the foundation of the U.S. laboratory response network and are the recipients of some of the recent biodefense funding, could be considered potential sources of surveillance data. Thus even if the tens of thousands of tests conducted in these laboratories each day failed to yield data that could be used for research purposes, they could be used to save lives and treat patients. Quality assurance tests could be used to monitor the data as necessary. In fact, global surveillance efforts would benefit from tighter links to all components of the clinical arena, including health care providers and physicians.

Because of the increasing opportunities for animal–human disease transmission resulting from globalization, a participant suggested that programs be established to encourage and facilitate the exchange of information between the animal and human disease surveillance communities. This information exchange would be of great benefit for disease detection, at least in the United States. Foot-and-mouth disease, for example, could be introduced into the United States with frightening ease, especially if it were done intentionally. Rapid detection, containment, and eradication would require shared intelligence between the animal and human disease surveillance communities.

Obstacles to Regional Surveillance:
The Caribbean Region as a Case Study

Development of the PAHO-administered Caribbean Surveillance System (CARISURV), based at the Caribbean Epidemiology Center in Port of Spain, Trinidad and Tobago, represents an attempt to regionalize infectious disease surveillance in the Caribbean. However, the system faces multiple challenges, both financial and organizational. For example, very little money is being spent on dengue surveillance, even though recent economic analyses suggest that the economic impact of dengue in the Caribbean exceeds that of the common cold. Perhaps one of the greatest challenges is that the Caribbean, like many developing regions, is a large area with diverse characteristics. It comprises about 35 countries whose people speak six different languages and have allegiances to different previous colonial powers.

Moreover, although most nations in the region are characterized as middle-income developing countries where public health and other problems are generally not as acute as in poorer countries, there are exceptions. Haiti's annual per capita GDP is about $700, the lowest in the hemisphere; other nations, such as Honduras, are also quite poor. Even among the so-called middle-income Caribbean countries, most governments lack sufficient resources to implement the public health measures that are considered their primary responsibility and for which they generally do not receive assistance from the private sector.

The region has very limited human resources devoted to the reporting of infectious diseases, and the statistics produced are notoriously unreliable. In most countries in the region, only a single person is responsible for reporting all infectious diseases, including HIV/AIDS. Laboratory capacity and technology support are also underdeveloped. This situation poses a great challenge for the region's foreign collaborators, including the United States. The capacity to conduct U.S. Food and Drug Administration–certified clinical trials for HIV vaccines in places such as Jamaica and Trinidad is limited by the fact that very few laboratories meet the criteria of the certifying agencies in the United States.

Strengthening of the regional surveillance capacity will require, among other things, the establishment of long-lasting training programs of the type described earlier in this chapter. Because there is a very limited number of trained personnel in the Caribbean—a situation typical of most countries in the developing world—training is extremely important for strengthening not just surveillance capacity, but also public health capacity in general.

Surveillance Success Stories

Although most observers would acknowledge the considerable challenges to meeting the need for an effective global surveillance system, there are some success stories that serve as good models for what can be achieved. The successes of polio and influenza surveillance efforts, for example, are attributed primarily to clear-cut goals and rewards (eradication, improved health for all). When attempts are made to enforce surveillance in places where there is no clear benefit—for example, where reporting creates a significant economic backlash—the challenges can be more difficult to overcome.

It was also pointed out that although the 1994 plague outbreak in India had a devastating economic impact, illustrating the negative global reaction that can result from sensationalized media reporting, few people are aware that India experienced another, more recent plague outbreak that was handled quietly, professionally, and appropriately. There was very little backlash in the form of international sanctions and the like. The pathogen was recognized, isolated, and confirmed within Indian laboratories using modern, state-of-the art resources; there was no need for international assistance. This success was due largely to extended collaborations with CDC and others aimed at improving India's surveillance and response capabilities.

INFORMATION AND COMMUNICATIONS TECHNOLOGY[9]

Workshop participants emphasized the potential of the Internet and the World Wide Web to change the way the work of public health is conducted, enabling enormous strides in the ability to understand, track, and fight infectious diseases. ProMED, e-mail, electronic chat rooms, the Global Outbreak Alert and Response Network (GOARN), and the Global Atlas of Infectious Diseases are just a few of the ways the Internet is being exploited for infectious disease control on a global scale. ProMED, for example, is a global public health information network that scans English, French, and Spanish media worldwide for reports of infectious disease outbreaks. Although not all ProMED reports are accurate, they allow investigations to begin more rapidly. Furthermore, ProMED reports are more public than country reports, and in many countries the press has a better surveillance capacity than the government. Reports can be obtained either by accessing the ProMED website or by subscribing to receive regular e-mails. (GOARN and the Global Atlas of Infectious Diseases are discussed below.)

Because the Internet and other communications technologies can be used to raise general awareness of the fundamental problems of global health, a participant suggested that they could also be used as leverage to ensure that those who can alleviate problems remain accountable—for example, governments that fail to provide resources for the Global Fund. Thus far, the groups that have used the Internet most effectively for such leverage have been targeting pharmaceutical companies, not governments.

Finally, although not discussed in detail during the workshop, telemedi-

---

[9]This section is based on the workshop presentations by Corber (2002) and Klaucke (2002).

cine was mentioned as a new, potentially very powerful tool. Telemedicine is the use of telecommunications technologies to deliver medical information and services when the provider and patient are separated by distance. It was suggested, for example, that recent advances in telemedicine may provide innovative solutions for improved screening of migrants. (See Chapter 2 for a discussion of migrant health.)

The Global Outbreak Alert and Response Network

In 2000, because the new International Health Regulations (IHRs) were not expected to be finalized and approved for another couple of years, WHO developed GOARN as the framework for some of the organizational activities necessary to be able to respond to urgent public health problems on a global level. GOARN is a technical partnership of 110 institutions and networks that work together to mobilize and pool resources for outbreak alerts and responses. Its purpose is to contain outbreaks by rapidly identifying, verifying, and communicating threats; to deliver appropriate technical assistance to affected areas; and to contribute to long-term outbreak preparedness.

GOARN is coordinated by a WHO operational team in Geneva, Switzerland, which works closely with WHO's six regional offices, 141 country offices, and liaison offices. The network's outbreak event management system has four main components: intelligence, verification, response, and follow-up. Information is gathered from various sources, both formal (e.g., WHO laboratory networks and regional and subregional networks) and informal (e.g., nongovernmental organizations and the media). The information is then verified by WHO offices and the countries involved, after which a risk assessment is conducted and the appropriate response determined. The appropriate response could include an investigation, preventive measures, case management, and/or the provision of information to the public.

Much (39 percent) of the information gathered by the network is transmitted to WHO from the Global Public Health Intelligence Network in cooperation with Health Canada. This real-time early-warning system scans more than a million Internet websites daily for news and other reports of infectious disease events. Other sources of intelligence include WHO (33 percent); ProMED (six percent); and various other sources, such as laboratories and nongovernmental organizations (22 percent).

To avoid the spread of rumors, information is not made available to the public until after it has been verified. Verification is a systematic process by which WHO confirms the occurrence of an outbreak, its etiology, and the need for assistance in an affected state(s). The network monitors only events of potential international public concern. The criteria used to determine whether an event is of international public concern include an unknown etiology, unexpectedly high morbidity or mortality rates, the need for assistance, the potential effect on international travel and trade, the current status of the outbreak relative to the IHRs, and any suspicion that the event was caused by an intentionally released biological agent.

Between March 2001 and March 2002, GOARN verified 195 events, most of which occurred in Africa (47 percent); some occurred in Asia and a very few in the Americas. The geographic distribution of the events reflects in part the quality of the public health infrastructure in these regions and the capacity to identify the events and respond appropriately at the national level.

The response component of GOARN involves providing rapid, appropriate, and effective assistance to the affected state(s); ensuring a level of response geared to the needs of the affected state(s); meeting daily to verify new intelligence and coordinate any responses; providing a field presence and coordination when needed; and maintaining systematic information management. From 1998 to 2001 there were more than 20 WHO-facilitated epidemic response missions, for which WHO was only one of several response partners. CDC, for example, was involved in more than half of these missions. All responses are tracked in a computerized outbreak event management system. WHO is currently developing a secure website for the network at which network members will be able to find timely information about ongoing responses.

Global Atlas of Infectious Diseases

The Global Atlas of Infectious Diseases is intended to be a web-based information and interactive mapping system that will support the global surveillance of infectious diseases. It will be used to provide access to infectious disease data and related information; standardized analyses of diseases, including maps, charts, and tables; a standardized dissemination mechanism; and an interactive data entry system for all partners.

At the website, one can find information about a disease in any particular area of the world or even a certain region within a larger geographic area. For HIV/AIDS, for example, one could select the African region of WHO and then find places where sentinel surveillance for HIV/AIDS was conducted for pregnant women in 1998. One could then select a particular country and locate the different sentinel sites within that country, or find a report identifying the sites by name. One could also develop charts that would enable comparisons across sites or over time, as well as link to other sources of information, such as epidemiology fact sheets for particular diseases.

REFERENCES

Barry M. 2002 (April 16). *Considering the Resources and Capacity for the Response.* Presentation at the Institute of Medicine Workshop on the Impact of Globalization on Infectious Disease Emergence and Control: Exploring the Consequences and Opportunities, Washington, D.C. Institute of Medicine Forum on Emerging Infections.

Cash R. 2002 (April 16). *Impediments to Global Surveillance and Open Reporting of Infectious Diseases.* Presentation at the Institute of Medicine Workshop on the Impact of Globalization on Infectious Disease Emergence and Control: Exploring the Consequences and Opportunities, Washington, D.C. Institute of Medicine Forum on Emerging Infections.

Cleghorn F. 2002 (April 16). *Considering the Resources and Capacity for the Response.* Presentation at the Institute of Medicine Workshop on the Impact of Globalization on Infectious Disease Emergence and Control: Exploring the Consequences and Opportunities, Washington, D.C. Institute of Medicine Forum on Emerging Infections.

Corber S. 2002 (April 16). *A Response to Shifting Threats.* Presentation at the Institute of Medicine Workshop on the Impact of Globalization on Infectious Disease Emergence and Control: Exploring the Consequences and Opportunities, Washington, D.C. Institute of Medicine Forum on Emerging Infections.

Demin A. 2002 (April 16). *Social Aspects of Public Health Challenges in a Period of Globalization: The Case of Russia.* Presentation at the Institute of Medicine Workshop on the Impact of Globalization on Infectious Disease Emergence and Control: Exploring the Consequences and Opportunities, Washington, D.C. Institute of Medicine Forum on Emerging Infections.

Gardner P. 2002 (April 17). *New Directions in Capacity Building.* Presentation at the Institute of Medicine Workshop on the Impact of Globalization on Infectious Disease Emergence and Control: Exploring the Consequences and Opportunities, Washington, D.C. Institute of Medicine Forum on Emerging Infections.

Gotuzzo E. 2002 (April 17). *The Global Application of Tools, Technology, and Knowledge to Counter the Consequences of Infectious Diseases: A Discussion of Priorities and Options.* Presentation at the Institute of Medicine Workshop on the Impact of Globalization on Infectious Disease Emergence and Control: Exploring the Consequences and Opportunities, Washington, D.C. Institute of Medicine Forum on Emerging Infections.

Gupta AR, Wells CK, Horwitz RI, Bia FJ, Barry M. 1999. The International Health Program: The fifteen-year experience with Yale University's Internal Medicine Residency Program. *Am J Trop Med Hyg* 61(6):1019–1023.

Henderson DA. 1998. Smallpox eradication—A cold war story. In: *World Health Forum.* Vol. 19. Baltimore, MD: Johns Hopkins School of Hygiene and Public Health. P. 113.

IOM (Institute of Medicine). 1985. *Vaccine Supply and Innovation.* Health Promotion and Disease Prevention. Washington, DC: National Academy Press.

IOM. 1987. *The U.S. Capacity to Address Tropical Infectious Disease Problems.* Report by a steering committee of the Board on Science and Technology for International Development. Washington, DC: National Academy Press.

IOM. 2005. *Scaling Up Treatment for the Global AIDS Pandemic.* Report by the Board on Global Health. Washington, DC: The National Academies Press.

Klaucke D. 2002. *Globalization and Health: A Framework for Analysis and Action.* Presentation at the Institute of Medicine Workshop on the Impact of Globalization on Infectious Disease Emergence and Control: Exploring the Consequences and Opportunities, Washington, D.C. Institute of Medicine Forum on Emerging Infections.

LeDuc J. 2002 (April 17). *The Global Application of Tools, Technology, and Knowledge to Counter the Consequences of Infectious Diseases: A Discussion of Priorities and Options*. Presentation at the Institute of Medicine Workshop on the Impact of Globalization on Infectious Disease Emergence and Control: Exploring the Consequences and Opportunities, Washington, D.C. Institute of Medicine Forum on Emerging Infections.

Miller M. 2002 (April 17). *Considerations for Shaping the Agenda*. Presentation at the Institute of Medicine Workshop on the Impact of Globalization on Infectious Disease Emergence and Control: Exploring the Consequences and Opportunities, Washington, D.C. Institute of Medicine Forum on Emerging Infections.

Netesov S. 2002 (April 17). *The Current Situation and Perspectives of International Collaboration in the Field of Biomedical Sciences: The Example of the State Research Center of Virology and Biotechnology, VECTOR*. Presentation at the Institute of Medicine Workshop on the Impact of Globalization on Infectious Disease Emergence and Control: Exploring the Consequences and Opportunities, Washington, D.C. Institute of Medicine Forum on Emerging Infections.

Paterson D, Swindels S, Mohr J. 1999 (Unpublished Data). *How Much Adherence is Enough? A Prospective Study of Adherence to Protease Inhibitor Therapy Using MEMSCaps*. Poster presented at 6th Conference on Retroviruses and Opportunistic Infections. Chicago, IL, Abstract 92.

Redfield R. 2002 (April 16). *Considerations for Drug Access and Delivery in the Developing World*. Presentation at the Institute of Medicine Workshop on the Impact of Globalization on Infectious Disease Emergence and Control: Exploring the Consequences and Opportunities, Washington, D.C. Institute of Medicine Forum on Emerging Infections.

Timperi R. 2002 (April 17). *Considerations for Shaping the Agenda*. Presentation at the Institute of Medicine Workshop on the Impact of Globalization on Infectious Disease Emergence and Control: Exploring the Consequences and Opportunities, Washington, D.C. Institute of Medicine Forum on Emerging Infections.

4

Creating a Framework for Progress

Globalization's emerging transnational social organization and epidemiological structure have transformed national public health into an international issue and necessitated the development of global health policy and governance. This chapter summarizes the workshop presentations and discussions on how sovereign states and nations must adopt a global public health mind-set. Also emphasized was the need for a new organizational framework to exploit the opportunities and overcome the challenges created by globalization and build the capacity needed to respond effectively to emerging infectious disease threats.

The trend toward increased funding for international health, such as that made available through the Global Fund to Fight AIDS, Tuberculosis, and Malaria (Global Fund) and President Bush's recently proposed Millennium Challenge Account (MCA), suggests that global public health is finally receiving the political attention it deserves, largely by virtue of its implications for economic development and national security. Global public health is no longer perceived as a costly charity endeavor; rather, it is increasingly being viewed as a cost-effective way of doing business, with countries poised to take action on selected diseases when there is an economic benefit to doing so.

Nonetheless, this increased funding and focus do not necessarily mean enough is being done collectively to enhance the global capacity to respond to either intentionally or naturally introduced infectious disease threats. As one workshop participant noted, global infectious disease control demands new approaches, and despite the welcome recent influx of funding, a fully coordinated and effective response will require even more money. Others admonished, however, that a lack of money should not be used as an excuse for not moving forward.

This chapter begins with a summary of the workshop discussion on the economic, national security, and other factors responsible for the changing perception of international health. This is followed by a summary of presentations and comments regarding some of the sources of and concerns about increased funding for international public health. The Global Fund and the MCA were discussed in some detail. The participants also briefly discussed the potential public health role of interim debt relief. Despite the promises of new funds and potential sources of even more funding, participants expressed many concerns, particularly with regard to how the funds would be used and whether they would be sustainable. Questions about the role of money also led to a brief discussion regarding the relative value of evidence-based public health and good governance.

With regard to the newer approaches required for global infectious disease control, several different but overlapping ideas were discussed. In addition to the need for consortia of financiers, such as the Global Fund, which are bigger and more flexible than individual agencies, most of the discussion focused on the need for public–private collaborations among states, interstate and regional organizations, nongovernmental organizations (NGOs), multinational corporations, and various other nonstate actors. Not only does the increasingly interconnected world provide opportunities for public–private collaborative responses on an international scale never before possible, but the intensifying cross-border traffic of microbes characteristic of globalization also demands that this opportunity be seized.

Greater interaction and fluidity between the developed and developing worlds, as exemplified by the bidirectional training programs discussed in Chapter 3, were also identified as a vital component of any effort to improve global public health. Throughout the workshop, participants discussed the most effective and sustainable ways to approach and manage collaborations with institutions, governments, and other partners in the developing world. Although some of these comments were included in the discussion of multinational research and training initiatives in Chapter 3, others are presented here.

Most of the public–private and other partnerships discussed during the workshop have been or are being designed to address the urgent and critical public health needs of the developing world and other countries with particular needs, such as Russia. Thus there was some discussion of the need to continue addressing U.S. domestic public health needs as well, especially the rise of antimicrobial resistance. Another important component of global public health identified by participants was the concept of public health as a global public good, especially with regard to product development and the dissemination of knowledge. The former was touched upon during the discussion on access to and delivery of antiretroviral agents in sub-Saharan Africa, as summarized in Chapter 3.

As globalization creates new governance challenges with respect to infectious disease prevention and control, the role of international law in infectious disease control policy has been shifting in important but uncertain ways. The chapter includes a summary of presentations on the revised International Health Regulations (IHRs) and the changing role of international law.

The chapter ends with a summary of the discussion pertaining to the need to study and understand the emergence of infectious disease threats within the larger social and political context. Historically, study of the emergence of infectious diseases has been restricted to the realm of biology. The political ecology of disease provides a new conceptual framework for understanding the public health consequences of globalization, including, for example, investment decisions that lead to environmental alterations, changing vector ecologies, and increased risk of the emergence and spread of infectious diseases.

THE CHANGING PERCEPTION OF INTERNATIONAL HEALTH[1]

A significant change in the perception of international health has occurred over the past decade. If asked 10 years ago to think about where international health dollars were being spent, most people would probably have thought of charity or the work of Mother Theresa or Albert Schweitzer. Today, international health is no longer perceived as a costly charity endeavor. Rather, as noted above, it is increasingly being perceived as a cost-effective investment with national security implications. The political and economic instability of sub-Saharan African countries with high HIV infection rates, for example, threatens the potential for strong international trade partnerships and poses a serious national security risk to the United States.

Although the renewed interest in international public health can be attributed mainly to economic and national security concerns, numerous other factors are at play. One participant described this renewed interest as a convergence of economic, humanitarian, and other ideals and strategic interests, including the following:

• Diplomacy—Public health is playing an increasingly important and constantly evolving role in international relations. Addressing the burden of

---

[1]This section is based on the workshop presentations by Adeyi (2002), Gardner (2002), Gordon (2002), and Patz (2002).

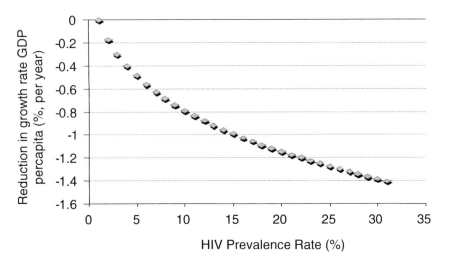

FIGURE 4-1   Impact of HIV on economic growth for 80 developng countries, 1990–1997.
SOURCE: The World Bank (2000).

disease in other countries by developing training and research programs, as described in Chapter 3, builds bridges of friendship and trust between U.S. and international scientists and fosters a deeper understanding and mutual respect between the United States and its partner nations. This represents a form of diplomacy with tremendous economic potential.

• Economic development—The global burden of infectious disease, which accounts for about 42 percent of the total global burden of disease, is not just about disease but also about money. The causal links among improved health status, an improved standard of living, and economic development are well established. The impact of HIV on economic growth in developing countries, for example, has been tremendous (see Figure 4-1). According to predictions by economist Jeffrey Sachs (WHO, 2000), if malaria had been eliminated 35 years ago, up to $100 billion would have been added to sub-Saharan Africa's 2002 gross domestic product of $300 billion. Because large-scale epidemics generally increase expenditures, reduce revenues, and raise the cost of doing business, businesses do what they can to minimize those impacts and avert lost productivity. Thus, for purely economic reasons, the private sector has taken a renewed interest in international public health, as have many governments. Unfortunately, increases in morbidity and mortality do not, by themselves, always tell a compelling story until the data are translated into economic terms. Money—not incidence and prevalence rates—is the language finance ministers and treasury secretaries understand.

• Increased opportunities for international trade—By investing in the public health systems of developing countries, the United States can develop valuable trading partners, thereby fostering its own economic growth.

• International political stability—Better health, improved economies, and stronger diplomatic relationships all foster stronger ties between the United States and its international partners and contribute to the latter's political stability.

• U.S. national security—Much of the renewed interest in global public health in the United States stems from concerns about national security. This was true even before the 2001 anthrax attacks. As one participant suggested, it is imperative for policy leaders and key decision makers to realize that global public health and infectious disease control are critical to preserving national and international economic and political security. In 1998, 200,000 people in Africa died in wars, and 2.2 million died from AIDS. In some countries, more than 30 percent of the military and 40 percent of teachers are infected with HIV. The national security implications of the growing global threat of infectious diseases were highlighted in a recent National Intelligence Council (NIC, 2000) publication, *The Global Infectious Disease Threat and Its Implications for the United States*.[2] The report contained several predictions and warnings, and since its publication, some of its predictions have clearly begun coming true:

— Infectious diseases are on the rise, and their potential costs are likely to be very high and far-reaching.

— Growing international concerns about infectious disease are likely to lead to travel- and trade-related frictions among countries.

— There is a growing risk of a bioterrorist attack against U.S. targets, both at home and abroad.

— HIV/AIDS will cause major demographic disruptions, perhaps to the point of undermining political stability in the poorest, hardest-hit, and most vulnerable countries.

— HIV infection rates among members of the armed forces are likely to be high enough that some militaries will be weakened and their ability to support U.S. peacekeeping missions limited.

---

[2]The primary responsibility of the National Intelligence Council, a U.S. government strategic think tank, is the production of long-term strategic intelligence analysis for the President of the United States and other members of the President's national security team. The report can be viewed online at http://www.cia/gov/cia/publications/nie/report/nie99-17d.html.

— Opportunities made available by advances in technology—Some cause for optimism comes from the existence of proven or promising technologies that can potentially be used for the prevention and control of infectious diseases. Vaccines, radiation therapy, and insecticide-impregnated bed nets are just a few examples.

— Confidence that comes from the recognition of past successes— Smallpox eradication demonstrated what global partnerships can achieve, given the necessary political will. The effort to control onchocerciasis in West Africa is another success story.

— Humanitarian concerns—The world is increasingly recognizing the inequity of a situation in which a tiny fraction of the world's population enjoys relatively robust health while the vast majority live from day to day with serious, avoidable morbidity and premature mortality.

— Improved U.S. public health—Lessening the burden of communicable diseases globally reduces the risks of importing diseases such as polio and tuberculosis (TB) into the United States. In addition, research advances made abroad often guide improvements in health care in the United States. The use of oral rehydration therapy (ORT) to treat the effects of severe cholera in overseas settings is an excellent example of how research advances abroad can lead to health improvements at home (i.e., the use of ORT to treat dehydration secondary to diarrhea, regardless of the cause). ORT is a low-tech scientific discovery that did not attract the notice of national research interests in the United States.

— The rule of law on a global level—One participant pointed out that most of the workshop discussion appeared to revolve around the notion of health as a humanitarian, economic, or national security goal. He called attention to the notion of health as an inalienable human right.

Thus for a number of reasons, infectious disease issues are being viewed as requiring a unified, global response despite differences in local interests. In March 2002, U.S. Senators William Frist and Jesse Helms announced plans to seek $500 million in additional funding for the fight against HIV/AIDS as part of the Bush Administration's emergency supplemental funding request for the war against terrorism and homeland security. In the Untied States, the need for international health expenditures is the subject of broad political consensus.

Likewise, to the extent that internationally agreed-upon goals, such as the development goals of the MCA, signify international consensus on the need to strengthen efforts to combat infectious diseases, such efforts are central to the global agenda as well. Public health is prominent among the MCA development goals, and infectious diseases are key elements of those public health goals. For example, one of the goals is to reduce by two-thirds the mortality rate among children under age five between 1990 and 2015. Another is to reverse the spread of HIV/AIDS, malaria, and TB.

However, the political attention that emerging infectious diseases are finally garnering does not necessarily mean that enough is being done collectively. For example, a number of countries are off track with regard to achieving a two-thirds reduction in the child mortality rate by 2015. This is especially true of the sub-Saharan African region, and of countries within other regions (including Eastern Europe and Central Asia, the Middle East and North Africa, and Southeast Asia) to varying degrees. This is not a country-specific or even a regional but rather a global concern.

INCREASED FUNDING FOR GLOBAL INFECTIOUS DISEASE CONTROL: SOURCES AND CONCERNS[3]

Although the renewed political commitment to international public health has led to increased funding for global infectious disease control, many workshop participants expressed concern regarding the sustainability of the funds, the realization of promised federal funding, the way the funds will be used, and whether the funds are sufficient to support the effort. According to 2001 estimates from the World Health Organization (WHO) Commission on Macroeconomics and Health, the price tag for new country-level programs, research and development, and the provision of other global public goods is $27 billion per year until 2007 and $38 billion per year by 2015. Current commitments total less than $7 billion.

Recent increased funds for global infectious disease control are coming largely from the U.S. government, for example, through greater expenditures on international health by the National Institutes of Health (NIH) and the U.S. contribution to the Global Fund. These funding sources are described below, along with President Bush's recently proposed MCA. In addition to their financial contributions to global infectious disease control, the Global Fund and the MCA exemplify the strong trend toward public–private partnerships within the context of global public health. Private-sector investments, such as funding from the Bill and Melissa Gates Foundation and Ted Turner's gift to the United Nations Foundation, have also contributed to the effort and are fueling a much greater awareness of the importance of these issues.

In addition to U.S. public and private investments, international organizations, such as Médecins sans Frontières (Doctors without Borders) and the Global Fund, are contributing to the effort. In fact, Europe and Japan each devote more of their gross national product to international health than does the United States.

---

[3]This section is based on the workshop presentations by Cash (2002), Gardner (2002), Kurth (2002), LeDuc (2002), Steiger (2002), and Widdus (2002).

NIH Funding

Although NIH funding for visiting overseas scientists has remained steady, direct foreign research awards have grown and are expected to continue to rise rapidly, and the foreign component of domestic NIH awards has risen about four-fold over the last six or seven years. Expenditures for NIH training grants are also beginning to increase slightly. In fiscal year 2002, overall NIH expenditures in the area of tropical infectious disease totaled $255,400,000. In late 2002, this figure was probably above the $300 million mark.

The Millennium Challenge Account[4]

On March 14, 2002, President Bush proposed the MCA—$5 billion of new and additional resources to complement the current bilateral assistance program of the U.S. Agency for International Development (USAID). The purpose of the MCA is to encourage greater responsibility and commitment by host governments to practice good governance, address social problems, and engage in a number of other efforts to improve their economy and standard of living. A number of criteria for eligibility and funding availability are being developed. The goal is to involve as many partners as possible, including the private sector.

The basic principle behind the MCA initiative is to shift from dispensing international assistance merely for geopolitical or political purposes toward directing resources to countries that have the greatest potential to make progress and the best policies in place, or to those whose policies the United States expects to change and improve over time. When the President announced the program, he enunciated three criteria for investment:

- Governance issues—Does the country have good policies in place for democracy, transparency, openness, and political participation?
- Investing in people—Does the country have, on its own, adequate policies for investing in education and health?
- Issues of economic freedom—Does the country have good macroeconomic and fiscal policies in place? What is its stance with regard to trade liberalization and privatization?

The program is in the process of developing a set of indicators for measuring a country's progress in terms of these criteria and, perhaps over time, translating this progress into eligibility to receive funding. This is

---

[4]Updated information on the MCA can be found at the website http://www.usaid.gov/mca/.

being done on an interagency basis, led by the U.S. Departments of State and Treasury and USAID. Program developers are seeking input on how to apply these three criteria and determine which countries are the most deserving of the additional assistance over and above what is provided by current international assistance programs, such as those of USAID and the U.S. Department of Health and Human Services (DHHS). The grants will be used as rewards for encouraging the development of good policies and making positive changes.

The decision to base the new grants on accomplishments rather than need was heavily influenced by work done at The World Bank showing that assistance has been effective in countries with better health policies and ineffective in countries with poor policies. A participant noted that the MCA represents an attempt to bring many of the issues discussed at the workshop into the arena of international development assistance in a way new to the U.S. government. In fact, the MCA and the Global Fund both serve as models for how the United States and perhaps other governments can revamp their models of foreign assistance in ways that better account for the role of public health in economic development.

At the same time, workshop participants raised some concerns about the proposed MCA. First, what impact will it really have on fighting infectious disease? The President has indicated that this is a general fund, not a health fund. By mentioning both health and education in his announcement, the President signaled that both sectors will receive substantial portions of the funds, but the amounts have not been determined. At this point, only an unspecified amount will be made available for HIV/AIDS and possibly other health concerns, such as TB and malaria. Moreover, while the scale of the MCA is quite significant compared with previous investments, and while the money to address these critical problems is potentially of enormous value, the details of implementation will ultimately prove the worth of the initiative.

It is important to note that, according to the President, the MCA will be independent of U.S. contributions to the Global Fund, and regardless of how the MCA is structured, the U.S. commitment to the Global Fund will continue. Whether the MCA is being created for humanitarian reasons or to serve U.S. interests, it reflects an increased appreciation for the importance of global health and the need for the United States to make real commitments to improving health in other parts of the world.

A second major concern regarding the MCA is the notion of performance-based funding. Globalization has led many to believe that capitalism works, that public health should learn from business, and that public health practitioners should operate in the same way as businesspeople. Although this may be true to a certain extent, some question whether public health practitioners should adopt the approaches of business throughout the international public health arena. The idea of performance-based funding has its positive aspects, and rewarding results is good practice. However, performance-based funding must not divert attention from the need to help those populations that have been failed by their governments.

The Global Fund to Fight AIDS, Tuberculosis, and Malaria

The concept of an international fund to fight HIV/AIDS, TB, and malaria was first proposed at the July 2000 Group of Eight (G8) Summit. By 2001, many governments and international agencies began discussing a variety of ideas for a global fund, including commodity purchase funds, advance-purchase commitment funds, broad health-sector interventions, funds for HIV/AIDS, and funds for a number of other specific diseases. Nothing crystallized, however, until May 11, 2001, when President Bush, along with the Secretary General of the United Nations (UN), announced that the United States would be the first donor to a global fund for HIV/AIDS, TB, and malaria.

The original contribution was $200 million. Since then the United States has increased its pledge to $500 million, including $200 million for fiscal year 2003. This commitment—about 25 percent of the $2 billion total pledged to date—represents by far the largest commitment by any government or institution to support the global fund concept.

Priorities of the Global Fund

When the President and the UN Secretary General announced the original commitment from the United States, the President outlined five principal priorities and emphases. As of this writing, the Global Fund has already achieved considerable progress toward meeting these five goals.

1. The Global Fund must be an independent, international public–private partnership, representing a new way of doing business and a new paradigm for foreign assistance. The United States and others had no interest in simply recreating the UN or even housing a new program within one of the UN agencies. Nor was the intent to divert attention from the important work done by the UN; rather, there was a frank recognition that there are limits to the work multilateral organizations as currently structured can do. In particular, there was a perceived need for a vehicle that would be attractive to both the nonprofit, nongovernmental private sector and the corporate private sector, as well as philanthropic organizations.

The Global Fund is incorporated as a nonprofit foundation under Swiss law. The governing board includes representatives of seven donor governments (the United States, Japan, the European Commission, Italy, France, the United Kingdom, and Sweden, the last three of which represent constituencies of smaller donors); seven developing-country governments, one from each of the seven WHO regions (Nigeria, Uganda, Brazil, Ukraine, Thailand, Pakistan, and China), plus an extra seat for Africa; and four private-sector entities, including an NGO from the northern hemisphere (a medical missionary organization from Germany), an NGO from the southern hemisphere (a community-based organization from Uganda), the Bill and Melinda Gates Foundation (which has contributed $100 million to the effort), and McKinsey and Company, which represents a broad coalition of for-profit private-sector actors. The private-sector representatives have been involved in structuring the Fund's secretariat, recruiting candidates for chief executive officer, and providing advice on the strategy and structure of the staff of the Fund. The board has four ex officio seats: The World Bank as trustee; WHO, which will be providing administrative support; the Joint United Nations Programme on HIV/AIDS (UNAIDS); and an additional NGO representing infected people and people affected by the three diseases.

The President intended the Global Fund to be a lean organization and a financial institution, not an implementing agency. It is a mechanism designed to move money to, not to operate, programs and partnerships. However, some internal functions will require personnel if the Fund is to achieve all of its goals.

Along with the notion of partnership, the intent was for the Global Fund to operate under a bottom-up approach. The Fund is not interested in dictating to countries how to spend their money or how to design their programs. Rather, countries are to inform the donors and international community of their priorities. During the current proposal process, the Fund is hearing about local needs and ways in which community organizations can work with their governments to develop and implement strategies.

2.   **The Global Fund should adopt an integrated approach.** A critical priority is to achieve a balance among regions, the three diseases, the prevention and treatment of each disease, and the care and support of those afflicted. Judging from the many proposals that have been recommended for funding thus far, the Fund has achieved a good balance; nevertheless, there is more work to be done.

3.   **The Global Fund must adopt a performance mind-set and be financially and programmatically accountable.** The Fund must ensure that the money is well targeted and well spent and that funded interventions have meaningful impacts on reducing morbidity and mortality. A key component of this goal is monitoring and evaluation of the Fund's performance over time.

4.   **The Global Fund will evaluate proposals through an independent technical review process.** The independent, impartial vetting of proposals by public health, scientific, and development experts is key to ensuring that

the Fund offers added value and is distinct from other organizations and institutions. In fact, the principle of technical review should set the Fund and its operations apart from most current efforts in the international arena.

The technical review panel currently comprises 17 experts from around the world, including the United States: six with expertise in HIV/AIDS, three with expertise in TB, three with expertise in malaria, and five with cross-cutting skills in the development and implementation of economic programs in other fields. The panel reviewed more than 330 proposals, nearly half from Africa, in mid-2002. After completing the review process, the panel referred a number of proposals to the board for its consideration.

5.   **The Global Fund should not be a lever for infringing on intellectual property rights.** The Fund must respect such rights and the need for innovation in the next generation of therapies and must find a way to respect international law and agreements within the context of the Doha Declaration.

March 2002 Global Fund Board Meeting

The Global Fund board members met in March 2002. Health and Human Services Secretary Tommy Thompson served as U.S. representative on the board; health ministers and ministers from most other governments involved were also present. The top item on the agenda was determination of the proposals to be funded, and the first grants were announced after the board met. The board also chose a chief executive officer.

In addition, the board discussed procurement policies and a framework for monitoring and evaluation. It finalized an agreement for the first phase of the initiative with The World Bank as the fund's trustee and the agreement with WHO as the provider of administrative support.

The Fund expressed its appreciation for the support, flexibility, and vision of Dr. Gro Harlem Brundtland, former Director-General of WHO, in creating a structure that allows the Fund to take advantage of the privileges of the UN system and save money by not recreating payroll systems, benefit systems, and pension programs; allowing the Fund's staff some of the diplomatic immunities and privileges of UN personnel; and giving the director and board broad latitude in hiring, firing, contracting, and making rules and regulations for its own internal operations.

Challenges of the Global Fund

Despite its success thus far, the Global Fund faces several challenges:

•   Monitoring and evaluation—The Fund must demonstrate success, not only because of the inherent value of showing the worth of this approach, but also to increase funding over time. The U.S. Congress and other legislatures around the world will be reluctant to provide additional money unless the Fund can demonstrate that it has done something different and has had a measurable impact in a relatively short amount of time. Deciding what is going to be measured, how it is going to be measured, and, ultimately, who is going to do the measuring poses an enormous challenge. Many of the Fund's donors recognize that money will have to be spent on monitoring and evaluation and that the Fund will need to acquire, either by contracting or by hiring staff, experts who know how to monitor grants on an ongoing basis and conduct evaluations ex post facto. Although the board is sympathetic to the idea that future funding of grants needs to be contingent on meeting performance targets, it is not clear what those targets are or how they should be measured.

• Procurement—A large number of applicants and successful proposal recipients intend to use Fund resources to purchase drugs and commodities. As this was the intent of the Bush Administration and donors, it poses no problem. However, recipients of the funding should respect certain principles regarding transparency, openness, and fairness of bidding, and they should base their purchase decisions on quality and sustainability, not just price. The board members have explicitly stated that they will not mandate any single methodology for procurement or the use of any particular agency to conduct procurement activities, nor will it list specific drugs or commodities to be considered for procurement. Local partners will be given the flexibility to inform the board regarding what they need to purchase and how. The board requests, however, that the purchasing occur within a rational framework.

• Proposal preparation, including potential assistance to countries and partnerships as they develop their proposals—The Fund learned some valuable lessons during the first round of proposal preparation, which occurred in a rather hasty manner. Most important, the Fund failed to provide enough clear information to partnerships and countries as they were preparing their applications, which contributed to the 50 percent rejection rate of proposals that did not meet the initial screening criteria for eligibility for future consideration. It was not clear who could submit proposals and how they should submit them, and there was a lack of involvement on the part of technical agencies, both bilateral and multilateral, in proposal preparation. DHHS, through the Centers for Disease Control and Prevention (CDC), provided technical assistance in the preparation of five or six proposals worldwide, although only one of these made it through the technical review process. Also, the number of proposals submitted far exceeded the Fund's expectations, and it was not ready to handle the more than 300 proposals it received. In the future, longer lead times for proposal preparation should be allowed, and much clearer and more explicit instructions on proposal preparation should be provided. The board needs to decide whether resources for planning grants should be invested up front or whether seed money should be provided to help partnerships prepare their proposals in a better way.

• Budgeting and investment strategy—The Fund had about $800 million in working capital for its first year. The amount available after that was uncertain. The board had to decide how to allocate resources among the recommended proposals and whether to make one year or multiyear commitments. If the entire $800 million were used during the first year and the availability of that same amount thereafter were uncertain, the Fund would be unable to plan for a second year of proposals. To honor its commitment to long-term funding, the Fund thus needs significantly more than $800 million.

• Economic and geographic balance—With regard to economic balance, the Fund has explicitly stated that it would like to focus on the poorest countries with the severest problems. Clearly, however, there are countries, such as Botswana, that have slightly higher incomes but still have terrible disease burdens. Many places in the world, such as the countries of the former Soviet Union, also face the potential for an explosion of epidemics but would be ineligible for aid if the Fund adopted a strict income scale. With regard to geographic balance, it is likely that the vast majority of the Fund's resources will be applied in Africa. However, the Fund does not want to neglect other parts of the world, such as the Caribbean, that also have significant problems deserving assistance, especially places where funding would be in the best interests of the United States.

• Achieving balance and establishing quotas—The Fund has set no guidelines for quotas for the prevention and treatment of AIDS, TB, and malaria and care for patients with these afflictions. Rather, the proposals dictate the priorities. Thus far, this has been a rational and reasonable approach. As the Fund moves forward, however, political pressure will likely lead to the setting of such quotas.

• Ceilings and floors for each proposal—The board has set neither lower nor upper limits on what a proposal can request. However, it has been recommended that the board consider setting such limits, as they would facilitate planning and budgeting over time.

• Involvement of the private sector—From the perspective of the Fund's administration, the one remaining task is to fully engage the private sector, including both for-profit and nonprofit organizations. It is generally believed that the Fund will not be sustainable over time without the commitment of nongovernmental entities, in terms of not just money, but also the design and implementation of proposals. There is still a great deal of skepticism and uncertainty within the private sector with regard to the Fund. In addition, the private sector was not fully engaged in the preparation of a number of proposals in the first round, and the partnerships created were not fully representative of nongovernmental and private-sector entities. The United States and its partners must work to ensure that the principle of partnership is fully applied. For this to occur, the for-profit sector must be comfortable with the Fund and recognize it as en entity with which it would like to do business.

Questions and Concerns About the Global Fund

As with the proposed MCA, workshop participants cited several concerns about the details and potential effectiveness of the Global Fund. One participant expressed discouragement that the Fund had already begun to review proposals and make some perhaps very significant awards in terms of funding without knowing what funding will be available in the future. Moreover, concern was voiced that appropriate criteria had not yet been put in place to evaluate success; that no ceilings had been set for proposals; and that no predetermined criteria had been established for distributing funds among AIDS, TB, and malaria. This issue is of particular concern with regard to the involvement of the private sector, which would likely be more supportive if these criteria were in place.

Thus the board did not make what are admittedly some difficult political decisions in January 2002, before announcing the first round of grant recipients. Although the United States has resisted pressure to award the funds quickly without addressing some of these important questions, others have been more willing to do so. Fortunately, however, in large part because of the excellent job done by the technical review panel, the proposals up for consideration, with one or two possible exceptions, are well conceived. The most costly proposals were eliminated during the review process because they were not well prepared and could not justify the amount of money being requested. Nonetheless, the future of the Fund is at risk if the board does not make the decisions discussed above.

Two of the board's immediate goals are to set ceilings and floors for proposal amounts and to develop a process for evaluating the financial accountability and absorptive capacity, as well as the programmatic quality, of approved proposals before the money is distributed. The board addressed ceilings and floors for proposals at a meeting held after the workshop. With regard to a process for evaluating financial accountability and absorptive capacity, as well as programmatic quality, it is too late to develop such a process from the perspective of the grant-making agencies. Nevertheless, carrying out that process before the first round of checks are cut will at least ensure that the process is in place before the second and third rounds.

Another concern with regard to the Global Fund relates to what many consider to be the inexcusably low 23 percent rate of implementation of directly observed treatment, short-course (DOTS). It was suggested that rectifying this situation should be one of the highest priorities in the awarding of funds, or even that some of the funds might be used to train scientists and physicians in how to influence political leaders, not just in the United States but also worldwide, with regard to the use of DOTS. In this connection, one participant noted that a number of the final first-round grants are for TB-related efforts, and one of the primary emphases of many of these efforts is the expansion of DOTS coverage.

One positive aspect of the Global Fund noted by a workshop participant was the emphasis on evidence-based public health. It was suggested that although there is considerable discussion of evidence-based medicine in the medical literature, there is far too little dialogue on the subject among the public health community. The long-term implications of certain practices often do not receive as much consideration as they should. That evidence-based public health is an important component of the Fund's priorities as part of the technical review and long-term evaluation processes is thus commendable (but see the summary below of the discussion of the value of evidence-based public health versus the need for good governance).

Other Possible Funding Sources for Global Infectious Disease Control

In addition to the above-described sources of new or increased funding for international public health, there are a variety of other potential funding sources, including international credit finance; domestic, nonpublic sources; and public budgets within countries, including debt relief. Of these, only interim debt relief was discussed in any detail during the workshop.

In contrast with traditional public finance, whereby government decides where expenditures should be made, interim debt relief funds go directly to the public treasury. It was suggested that the stream of income from debt relief received by a country over a period of several years can significantly increase the country's public budget and, if used appropriately, can also significantly benefit its public health. Indeed, a participant noted that at a recent UN General Assembly meeting, member states agreed that a portion of debt relief monies must be used to address health issues. While developing their plans for spending their debt relief monies, recipient nations must designate how they will spend the funds in the health sector. The general goal is to use the funds to build public health infrastructure, and to ensure that there is a health component to the debt reduction plan as well. On the basis of preliminary data from The World Bank, some of the approximately 32 countries recently eligible for interim debt relief are planning to increase their health expenditures by about 25 percent per year, depending on how much money they receive.

Already in Madagascar and Cameroon, for example, significant sums of money from debt relief have been channeled into health, particularly for new HIV/AIDS resources. The same thing has happened elsewhere, for example, in Chad, Burkina Faso, and Malawi. In total over the past several years, an additional $36 million annually has been allocated for health in some nine or 10 countries, depending on how the scope of the health sector is defined.

At the same time, several factors will determine whether this source of funding is actually going to make a difference. First, success will require that the recipient nation have a strong central political commitment to health, with a champion other than the prime minister or minister of finance, who is more likely to use debt relief funds for roads or agriculture. Second, the recipient nation should be very specific about where the funds will be directed. In Cameroon, for example, recent interim debt relief funds were targeted specifically at interventions for high-risk transmitters of HIV, including the military. Finally, the recipient state should be able to anticipate the difficulties associated with spending money rapidly. In Cameroon, for example, although the amount of money was not large in absolute terms, it was much larger than what the country had been accustomed to. Considerable effort was required to use the money effectively.

Answers Other Than Money

Despite the clear call for more funds and greater flexibility in how those funds are used, many workshop participants agreed that money is not a cure-all. They warned that funding must not become an overriding issue in the discussion of what steps need to be taken next with regard to the prevention and control of emerging and reemerging infectious diseases on a global scale.

As one participant argued, funding global infectious disease control is not just a matter of doing more; it is also a matter of doing better and channeling external assistance where it will make a significant difference. Care must be taken to spend the money well and to consider the capacities of countries and agencies to absorb it. In the past, aid that has been well targeted has been well spent. When funds have been channeled to places where the disease burden is high and where there are reasonably good policies in place or prospects for changing bad ones, the money has generally been used to good purpose. This contrasts with situations in which the money has been spent purely for narrow political or geopolitical reasons. Nor should the world be diverted by this large sum of money from funding other ongoing programs that are already making a difference.

Other workshop participants agreed that simply putting money into problems is not necessarily going to solve them. First, problems need to be identified and delineated; this often requires strengthening basic research capacity. The money then needs to be targeted accordingly. For example, it is not necessarily enough to know that pathogens are being distributed around the world in the wheel wells of airplanes. Growing evidence suggests that only certain types of pathogens, such as the Spanish strain of *Streptococcus pneumoniae*, are in fact spreading globally. This raises the question of what makes the Spanish strain of this bacterium so globally adept. As another example, salmonellosis in general is not necessarily the problem in the United States, but a specific strain that is resistant to five drugs (although there was some disagreement on this point).

One participant acknowledged that insufficient funding can kill a project but noted that most successful international collaborations with developing countries have not been contingent on access to additional money. The amount of money needed to conduct the task at hand is usually not enormous and should not be seen as an obstacle to moving forward. Others disagreed on this point, however.

Another participant suggested that, because globalization is not necessarily something new, but rather changing in its degree and pace, the fundamental problems of public health have not changed. The biggest issue is still a lack of resources—not just those required to research new products, but also the tens of billions of dollars needed to get existing products into use and to strengthen health system management in the poorest countries. The funding needed to address these underlying problems should not be underestimated, and care must be taken not to let aspects of globalization that exacerbate public health problems detract from meeting this need.

Some participants expressed concern that too great an emphasis on evidence-based public health, as is the case with the Global Fund, could deflect attention from underlying problems that play a more fundamental, etiological role in the growing global threat of emerging and reemerging infectious diseases. For example, the implementation of DOTS is not necessarily a matter simply of applying evidence-based public health. Perhaps more important, good governance is a prerequisite for employing any kind of public health, evidence based or not, in the fight against emerging and reemerging infectious diseases, as the current public health situation in Russia illustrates.

With regards to DOTS, one of the greatest problems faced by Russia is the sheer political complexity of implementing such a program on a large scale in a country that has its own, very different established practices and institutions. The implementation of DOTS on a countrywide scale is not an exercise or technical challenge per se; it has more to do with transactions and bargaining. For many reasons, including the fact that the country had its own way of doing things in the Soviet era, Russia has as yet not officially adopted DOTS as either a treatment or a diagnostic approach. To move from the point where Russia is today—with respect to not only DOTS but also other outdated or unscientific means of diagnosis and treatment—to the point where leading Russian scientists are collaborating with their partners in other parts of the world and adopting internationally recognized practices will require a dialogue with local institutions and interest groups that were trained under and are comfortable with the old system. Recent discussions in Moscow offer hope that progress is being made in this direction.

Although Russia is making progress, good governance is proving a much more difficult task in other parts of the world. It was noted that in the Middle East, for example, only one government truly exercises democracy; other governments, which often distort the Islamic religion for political purposes, are not accepted by their populations. One participant pointed out that to establish public health systems in the Middle East that are functional and efficacious in the long term, it will be necessary to encourage the other countries in the region to accept democracy.

Good governance must precede any large-scale effort to improve the public health system. The Republic of South Africa, for example, needs good governance to influence NGOs involved in the distribution of HIV/AIDS drugs to the neediest populations. As another example, public health is virtually nonexistent in the Democratic Republic of Congo, where, not surprisingly, so many reemerging infectious diseases originate. But how should good governance be established? It is essential that American or European public health strategies not be imposed in other parts of the world without modifications appropriate to local conditions. (The issue of governance was also discussed within the context of the changing role of international law in the global public health arena, as summarized at the end of this chapter.)

THE ROLE OF PUBLIC–PRIVATE PARTNERSHIPS[5]

One of the recurring themes of the workshop was the vital role of public–private partnerships in building the global capacity to prevent and control emerging and reemerging infectious disease threats, whether intentionally or naturally introduced. It was noted that the Global Fund, as described earlier in this chapter, reflects this new spirit of partnership in a unique way. Not since the founding of the United Nations Children's Fund (UNICEF) 50 years ago has the world seen the creation of an entity with so

---

[5]This section is based on the workshop presentations by Adeyi (2002), Cash (2002), Cleghorn (2002), Fidler (2002), Kimball (2002), Klaucke (2002), Kurth (2002), Leaning (2002), and LeDuc (2002).

much potential in the international health arena. A number of other, similarly promising partnerships have also recently been formed, including the Global Alliance for Vaccines, Stop TB, UNAIDS, and the International AIDS Vaccine Initiative. In addition, CDC's Framework for Progress strategy, discussed in detail below, places a heavy emphasis on partnership. WHO also has a number of new partnerships with private industry, in addition to its many traditional partnerships with laboratories, ministries of health, and universities. For example, the WHO program Roll Back Malaria involves working with oil companies (e.g., ExxonMobil and Eni) to extend medical assistance to surrounding communities in the countries in which they operate; with mining companies (e.g., Placer Dome and World Alliance for Global Health, BHP Billiton) to spray insecticides to stop the spread of malaria among employees and their families; and with tourist hotels (Zimbabwe Sun and Kenya Hotel Association) to spray insecticides and apply other measures to reduce the incidence of malaria in communities.

Public–private partnerships are a conduit for providing critical treatments for disease in countries where so many people still lack access to such treatments. The arrangements are most useful in situations in which complementary skills are needed to solve otherwise intractable problems. As one participant described them, public–private partnerships tackle problems that are otherwise not being addressed, are globally important, are historically intractable, disproportionately affect the poor, perpetuate poverty, and require the skills of both the public and private sectors.

Moreover, today's public–private initiatives serve as potentially valuable social experiments. It is hoped that by examining their progress over the next 10–20 years, the most effective way for such partnerships to operate can be determined.

The key way to obtain the best return on the dollar is the establishment of public–private partnerships that are long-lasting, that is, that endure longer than a funding cycle of one, two, or even five years. Such partnerships can build capacity over the long term. A participant noted that the partnerships developed by the U.S. armed forces worldwide are a model for success: they have very long funding cycles, they build capacity over the long term, and they include collaborators in developing countries as equals. Another participant suggested that the U.S. government's long-term narcotics-fighting and customs partnerships in the Caribbean can be instructive. The U.S. Customs Service has formed such partnerships to stem the tide of illegal drugs coming from the Caribbean into the United States. U.S. personnel travel to the Caribbean countries to train their personnel and influence local systems. The Pan American Health Organization–administered Caribbean Epidemiology Center is trying to apply this same approach in its management of HIV/AIDS.

Although public–private partnerships are an important trend, they are not a panacea. In fact, like money, they often detract from dealing with the root causes of public health problems and from holding accountable those who should be addressing those problems. Public–private collaborations cannot substitute for governments, both rich and poor, that properly fulfill their responsibilities to build and maintain the necessary public health infrastructure and ensure that their citizens receive proper health care services.

A participant noted that the use of these partnerships in a global effort to improve public health capacity requires adoption of a bottom-up, grass-roots approach whereby all agencies, organizations, and persons involved maintain a global mind-set and focus on how they can work together to better address the many issues they must confront. On the other hand, with no effective "global government" or feasible means of top-down implementation, the question arises of how to orchestrate a bottom-up approach that encourages entrepreneurial action on the part of thousands of different agencies. One of the largest obstacles to a global response is its management.

Types of Public–Private Partnerships

A participant suggested that, to avoid making broad, inaccurate generalizations about how public–private partnerships form and why they work, it would be helpful to define "public," "private," and "public interest" and clarify whether public goods can come from private products. The Initiative for Public–Private Partnerships and Health, which has recently been studying these issues, has defined three basic components of the public and private sectors on the basis of who owns the assets under discussion: the public sector, civil society, or for-profit organizations (see Figure 4-2). If the organization is based on state-owned assets, it is part of the public sector, which includes both governmental agencies and intergovernmental agencies such as WHO. If the organization is based on assets that are not state owned, it is either a civil-society or for-profit organization. Some of the former tend to define themselves by what they are not, that is, NGOs. Others are academic institutions, which receive money from the public sector but are still essentially private unless they are state universities, philanthropies, or other nonprofit organizations. For-profit organizations include pharmaceutical companies, biotechnology companies, and other commercial, non–health-sector companies.

These organizations can collaborate and interact in numerous ways, resulting in many different modes of operation. In developing countries, for example, NGOs have traditionally collaborated with governmental organizations in the delivery of health care services. Also, both health-related and non–health-related industry organizations conduct activities in the interest of health or other social concerns, whether related to their core business or not. For example, GlaxoSmithKline, in response to concern about teenage

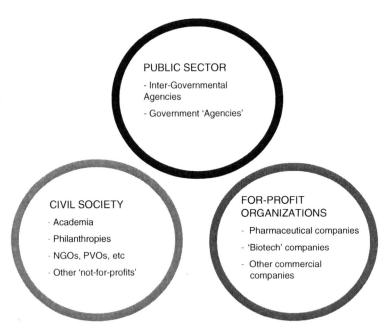

FIGURE 4-2   Components of the public and private sectors.
SOURCE: Widdus (2002).

suicide in Eastern Europe, started supporting hotlines so teenagers could talk about their problems; ExxonMobil funds the Medicines for Malaria Venture, a public–private partnership dedicated to the development of new antimalaria drugs; a South African power company, Eskom Enterprises, supports AIDS prevention efforts; and Apple Computer has, through various programs, donated both hardware and software to educational institutions.

Where the secretariats of these collaborations are located is an important issue, since a partnership tends to operate according to the rules of the secretariat's organization or host institution. Thus many partnerships, such as the Global Alliance for Vaccines and Immunization and Roll Back Malaria, are more strictly public-sector programs with private-sector participants. When the pharmaceutical industry is represented by only one member of a board of 18 people, for example, the collaboration is not essentially a joint venture.

Public–private interactions among organizations range from more traditional relationships that involve grant giving and receiving and the procurement of goods and services to some newer modes of interaction, including privatization of the delivery of health services, with the public sector setting and monitoring the rules and quality of service. This new type of interaction is occurring more frequently in both developed and developing countries, contrary to the popular notion that governments are the primary providers of health care services in the latter. In India, for example, 80 percent of the population receives health care services from private providers.

Joint Venture Partnerships

Another type of nontraditional public–private interaction that is becoming increasingly common is the achievement-oriented joint venture partnership. Its attributes include:

- A shared objective agreed upon by all participants, even though their motivations and values may differ.
- Shared risk taking, which has become inherent in new ways of doing business and can lead to innovation.
- Shared decision making, without which there is not a true partnership.
- Contributions from each participant.
- Benefits to each partner, although these may differ.

About 70 international partnerships with these attributes are involved in health research, health care, and health care delivery. These include partnerships that generate basic knowledge in the area of health (e.g., genomics) and are funded by private industry but involve government agencies and private universities; product development partnerships; collaborations that involve the delivery of donated, discounted, or subsidized products; partnerships that strengthen health services, especially in areas where AIDS is endemic and where health services must be strengthened to ensure the proper use of the products that are delivered; education partnerships; product quality or regulation improvement partnerships; and various broadly coordinated, multifaceted efforts.

Approximately 40 of these 70 partnerships are involved in the development and delivery of donated products (including drugs, vaccines, diagnostics, contraceptives, vector control agents, and devices and equipment) in the poorest countries, which generally lack the financial and public health infrastructural resources for product delivery. Examples include the Concept Foundation (contraceptives), the International Trachoma Initiative, the Botswana Comprehensive HIV/AIDS Partnership, and the Mectizan Donation Program (river blindness). A significant proportion of deaths from infectious diseases that occur in the poorest parts of the world are preventable by cheap, satisfactory, off-patent medications that exist but are inaccessible to people disadvantaged by poverty and a weak public health infrastructure. In fact, the approximately 300 WHO-listed "essential" drugs never make it to 50 percent or more of the world's population (see Figure 4-3). A smaller fraction of these deaths are caused by a lack of access to new products, such as AIDS medications and treatments for drug-resistant malaria and TB, which are considered too costly to introduce into low- and middle-income developing countries, where prospects for a return on such an investment are poor. A price concession is usually necessary for new products to be introduced at the earliest possible opportunity.

These collaborations generally address any and all aspects of product development and delivery, from the initial research phase to product introduction. Thus, collaborators from different partnerships often face similar challenges with regard to conducting clinical trials, managing intellectual property, devising a plan for product introduction, conducting market assessments, and a variety of other tasks. These partnerships are also continually evolving; some partnerships currently involved in delivering donated drugs originated as research collaborations. One of the goals of the Initiative for Public–Private Partnerships for Health is to foster the exchange of knowledge and information among these many partnerships, which usually are legally independent or work separately. For example, collaborations that are only now addressing basic research questions can learn from other partnerships that have previously worked on similar issues.

Partnerships Involving Nongovernmental Organizations

Because the globalization of infectious diseases requires a highly coordinated and yet highly diversified response on the part of many public- and private-sector partners, it was suggested that the U.S. public health community and government tap the expertise of NGO leaders. NGO humanitarian responders have become increasingly important over the past decade in serving as the focal point for the implementation of foreign aid. They can also serve as a good source for ideas, collaborators, and colleagues. They form an international community that includes many young Americans who are funded by U.S. government grants; they have a good understanding of the issues in infectious disease and globalization; they are improving prevention and surveillance capacities and are sensitive to issues of human rights and international law; they have a good sense of public health priorities and population-level needs; and they have developed laudable processes for standards setting, accountability, outcome evaluation, and strengthening of institutions.

Twinning

It was suggested that the U.S. public health community should consider the potential role of twinning, an arrangement that involves matching sister

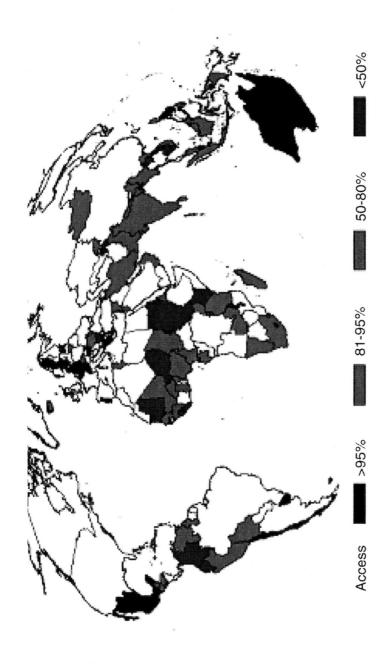

Access   ■ >95%   ■ 81-95%   ■ 50-80%   ■ <50%

FIGURE 4-3   Many people still lack access to essential drugs.
SOURCE: WHO (2003).

cities or organizations or institutions from different cities so they can share expertise, transfer technologies, enhance their surveillance capabilities, and generally assume responsibility for each other. The practice has become very popular in Europe and appears to provide a realistic solution to ensuring that local needs are met while being tied to a greater international network of needs. In Germany, for example, prisons are twinning in an effort to fight the rise of TB among the prison population. Also in Europe, countries themselves are twinning. Germany is twinning its public health sector, including its insurance system, with that of Poland; many similar efforts are being undertaken as a way to prepare countries in Eastern Europe to join the European Community. Twinning, however, is still a relatively undeveloped idea in the United States.

Involving Multinational Corporations in Global Public Health

Given the obvious role of multinational corporations in public–private partnerships, workshop participants discussed at length how to engage the interest of these companies more fully in global infectious disease control. The question was raised of what incentives exist for multinationals to maintain healthy workforces and otherwise contribute to dealing with global public health crises. As one of the strongest sectors of global society, multinational corporations could potentially make a tremendous contribution to efforts to improve global health. This is especially true in countries that lack the necessary infrastructure, for example, those where DOTS does not exist. Workshop participants cited several challenges that must be overcome if multinational corporations are to be recruited for this purpose:

• The fluctuating nature of business makes it difficult to maintain alliances with the private sector over time. Even though in 1996, when the Asia-Pacific Alliance was established in an effort to include multinationals in the fight against AIDS, corporations were generally receptive to being involved in promoting AIDS prevention, that receptiveness did not necessarily last. The reality is that business cycles up and down, leadership changes, and priorities within the corporate culture do not always include the company's continuing that type of underwriting.

• Cultural divides make it difficult to institutionalize public health practices in transnational corporations that are operating in multiple cultures. For example, there is a strong reluctance to impose in other countries workplace policies that would be considered appropriate in the United States, especially with regard to HIV-related programs.

• Issues of intellectual property rights can slow progress. The tension between intellectual property rights and access to drugs illustrates a fundamental difference between the interests of multinational corporations and those of the global public health system. In particular, pharmaceutical companies want to protect their highly lucrative markets, for example, against cheap antiretroviral agents available from other parts of the world.

• The notion that it is not the responsibility of private companies to provide public goods can also slow progress. Companies that are increasingly being asked to participate in public–private partnerships or to fund public health efforts typically respond by arguing that public health is a public good and should be the responsibility of the governments of the developing countries where the problems exist. Many argue that it is both unfair and unsustainable to ask for a public good from private enterprises.

• Some believe that small businesses should play a role. Although the responsibility of transnational corporations may be more apparent, about 80 percent of employed people worldwide work for small to medium-sized businesses, many of which are involved in international trade. In many countries, moreover, the informal trade sector is actually much larger than the formal trade sector, and some would argue that these other, smaller enterprises also have a responsibility.

• The communication gap between the public health system and the private sector can make it difficult for the two to work together. If inappropriate trade restrictions were to be imposed on a country because of an outbreak of an infectious disease, for example, public health officials could assist the private sector by providing information on why a product posed no threat of transmitting the disease.

• There is a need for a new economic model that would provide incentives for multinational corporations to participate, especially given the competing priorities unrelated to infectious disease within both individual companies and the larger market. It is unclear what such a model should or could entail.

Creative strategies are thus needed to address misaligned incentives, encourage the commercial sector to participate in global public health efforts, and build bridges between the NGO and corporate sectors. Some participants commented that devising such strategies will be extremely difficult. Others noted, however, that several groups, such as the World Economic Forum and the International Chamber of Commerce, are encouraging business programs to combat infectious diseases, including HIV/AIDS, TB, and malaria, and some strategies that are already known may be worth examining or revisiting.

For example, it might be possible to learn from examining the histories of companies that have long provided health care for their employees, as was done during the era of plantation medicine. Likewise, several ongoing case studies are examining the role of the private sector in global public health. For example, if the cease-fire and agreements in Angola continue to hold, the United States and other governments will continue to put considerable pressure on the major oil companies to play a more positive role in the country's reconstruction and to move from the cities into long-neglected rural areas. As another example, Anglo American, a global leader in mining and natural resources, recently decided not to comply with the recommendation of an in-house feasibility study to provide free antiretroviral therapy to its HIV-positive employees in South Africa. The HIV incidence rate among the company's workforce is estimated to be 20 percent, but there were concerns about sustainability and how free antiretroviral therapy would fit into the overall position of the country on the treatment of HIV/AIDS. This kind of enlightened self-interest on a company's part can create a dual system whereby company employees have substantially greater access to health care than the general population. The company intends to engage in discussions with other major companies in South Africa, as well as the South African government, before moving forward.

A participant suggested that the diverse market interests of different companies could be exploited to provide opportunities for improving global public health in some basic ways. For example, Procter & Gamble, a large transnational manufacturer of consumer products, produces a number of items, such as soap, that are relevant to public health. The company could make soap available at low cost to a market of billions of people around the world who have very limited economic power. Other companies could do the same with safe drinking water. Although bottled water is a large industry in developed countries, it is too costly for most of the populations in need in developing countries. Other water treatment products may be more affordable, and the companies that make these products could participate in efforts to provide cheap, safe drinking water. In response to this suggestion, however, a participant noted that this kind of business philanthropy is quite different from the enlightened self-interest that motivates a company to seek to preserve a healthy workforce. It is important to recognize that companies, regardless of what business they are involved in, have motivations very different from those of health care agencies.

A participant suggested that interactions with multinationals be focused at the early stages of investment, when business decisions are first made. For example, if a company moving into an area could configure itself or the way it does business so as to lower the incidence of AIDS among its workers, this might be more effective than waiting until a treatment approach is the only choice. This point speaks to the general question of what the commercial sector can do so that bad health is not an adverse outcome of development. Preproject health assessments may provide at least a partial solution.

Preproject Health Assessments

When companies move into new areas, they usually conduct cost–benefit assessments, which typically include environmental assessments whose results are presented in environmental impact statements. Likewise, when considering loaning or guaranteeing money for certain infrastructure projects or the facilitation of foreign investment in other countries, The World Bank and U.S. government agencies, such as the Overseas Private Investment Corporation, are starting to use highly sophisticated and extensive environmental assessment rules to make their decisions. It was suggested that the public health community might benefit from examining this environmental model and evaluating the extent to which health issues could be addressed by this type of proactive approach.

A public health assessment would benefit not only the health of the workforce and potentially that of the general public, but also the company's productivity and economic profit. If a particular decision were not cost-effective, it would be extremely difficult to convince a company to make that choice in the interest of either the health of the workforce or general public health. On the other hand, if an assessment predicted that a particular decision would cause an increased incidence of malaria in the workforce, which in turn would lead to decreased productivity, it would be in the company's best interest not to make that choice.

One participant expressed concern that environmental impact statements often accomplish nothing other than generating paper and employing consultants who have a vested interest in affirming the decision already made by a company. The potentially negative long-term environmental impacts of a project often are not reflected in the statement. Disease impact statements would likely by plagued by the same problem. Nevertheless, even the developing world has expended a great deal of effort on environmental issues, and in so doing has captured the imaginations of many populations and effectively sent the message that they must preserve their environment. The public health community has never captured anyone's imagination in quite the same way. Perhaps there is something to be learned from the environmental movement.

Industry as an Educational Resource

A few participants commented on the innovative roles that private industry could potentially play in global infectious disease control. When people seek help from the pharmaceutical industry, they usually ask for money or products, not intellectual or educational capacity. Industry can, however, provide the latter resources and in so doing, serve as a partner in global health. For example, a multifaceted collaboration involving the public health community and the pharmaceutical and communications industries could provide a powerful opportunity to address the emergence of drug-resistant pathogens.

A major cause of multidrug resistance is a lack of adherence to recommendations for the proper use of medicines. The pharmaceutical industry and public health community have a mutual interest in addressing this problem, and the global communications industry could provide the means to do so. This kind of effort would be especially helpful in developing countries, where there are fewer educational resources in general and where the challenges to maintaining high rates of adherence to therapies, particularly DOTS and antiretroviral therapy, are great. Some efforts along these lines have recently been made in the United States, including the distribution of educational materials on antimicrobial resistance from CDC and the American Medical Association by pharmaceutical company sales representatives. As another example, the secretary of Health and Human Services recently announced a new program whereby pharmaceutical company sales representatives will be distributing educational materials on anthrax, smallpox, and other potential bioterrorism agents.

The Centers for Disease Control and Prevention's Framework for Progress: An Emphasis on Partnerships

For public health workers, the global movement of people, animals, and goods and the concomitant movement of diseases across national borders has always been a fact of life, and CDC has long engaged in efforts to prevent and control infectious diseases beyond the borders of the United States. In recognition of the accelerating pace of globalization, CDC has prepared a document, *Protecting the Nation's Health in an Era of Globalization: CDC's Global Infectious Disease Strategy*, which is meant to serve as a framework for enhancing, consolidating, and focusing CDC's efforts to prevent and control infectious diseases on a global scale. The document begins by stating, "it is not possible to adequately protect the health of our nation without addressing infectious disease problems that occur elsewhere in the world" (CDC, 2002, p. 6). The strategy places a strong emphasis on partnerships.

In preparing the document, the authors drew on many sources, including previous reports of the Institute of Medicine. In addition to extensive internal review of the document, comments from experts were solicited at a November 2000 meeting in Atlanta, Georgia. The strategy, released at the International Conference on Emerging Infectious Diseases, held in Atlanta in March 2002, identifies six priority areas, described below.

1. **International outbreak assistance.** In hospital wards, refugee camps, villages, and almost every other setting where outbreaks occur, CDC has built a reputation for providing expert technical assistance in identifying and controlling risk factors for disease transmission. Rather surprisingly, CDC's international outbreak assistance has been provided largely ad hoc, with little long-term planning, dedicated funding, or ability to provide follow-up assistance after the acute emergency response.

Outbreaks offer unique opportunities to learn more about the dynamics of disease transmission; the effectiveness of prevention, control, and treatment strategies; and the risk factors for severe and fatal disease. Because of the public nature of disease outbreaks, they also offer opportunities to bring organizations together. Knowledge gained in one investigation can often be applied to other situations, including those within the United States.

Thus, one of the underlying principles of CDC's global infectious disease strategy is that international outbreak assistance is an integral function of CDC, as opposed to an ad hoc activity. To take full advantage of the opportunities offered by international outbreak investigations, CDC must have targeted resources and an enhanced capacity for laboratory and epidemiological investigations, as well as the ability to offer support for follow-up activities, including surveillance and the development, implementation, and evaluation of long-term preventive measures.

2. **Global approach to disease surveillance.** Accurate information about emerging infectious diseases must travel at least as rapidly as the diseases themselves, which in this day of jet travel is quite rapid indeed. To remain one step ahead of multiple epidemic waves, public health authorities worldwide are increasingly relying on modern, rapid laboratory diagnostics; electronic connectivity; and communications networks.

Despite the many and real obstacles to global surveillance (see Chapter 3), some progress has been made. Many global surveillance networks exist, including both those that are disease specific, such as the WHO Global Polio Laboratory Network, and those that are regional. Notable progress has been achieved at the regional level; examples include the Amazon and southern cone networks in South America (see Chapter 3). Many of these regional networks are supported through CDC partnerships.

However, a global approach to disease surveillance will require that in the long run, regional and disease-specific networks expand, interact, and evolve into a global network of networks. WHO has assumed a leadership role in organizing this effort, of which CDC is a critical component.

3. **Applied research on diseases of global importance.** Several years ago, one could easily have argued that understanding the complex ecology of the West Nile virus was neither an appropriate nor a high priority for

CDC, as the virus did not affect U.S. citizens to any great degree. The introduction of West Nile virus into New York City and its subsequent spread throughout the eastern United States changed that perception and highlighted the value of conducting applied research not just on diseases that occur in the United States, but also on those that are globally important. Indeed, experience gained by CDC personnel while investigating an outbreak of West Nile virus in Romania in the mid- to late 1990s helped ensure that CDC virologists, entomologists, and epidemiologists would be familiar enough with the disease to recognize it early in the course of the New York City outbreak and provide informed advice for prevention strategies.

The breadth and depth of CDC's laboratory and epidemiological capacities are critical resources. CDC's global infectious disease strategy argues that it is in the best interest of the United States to maintain and strengthen that capacity through an active program of applied research on diseases of global importance.

4. **Application of proven public health tools.** To carry out its mission, CDC must engage in implementation research that translates science into meaningful differences in the rates of morbidity and mortality from infectious diseases on a global scale and in a timely manner. A good example of the kind of proven public health tool addressed by this priority area is the insecticide-impregnated bed net, which has been shown in many field trials to reduce rates of morbidity and mortality from malaria. Yet despite this knowledge, the bed nets are used by less than 10 percent of people at risk. There are many other underutilized but proven public health tools, such as auto-disable (one-use) syringes to prevent bloodborne transmission of hepatitis B and C viruses and HIV, point-of-use chlorination and safe water storage to prevent waterborne diseases, routine immunization with vaccines for hepatitis B and other diseases, and single-dose therapy to prevent perinatal HIV transmission.

Each of these tools is underutilized for slightly different reasons, although there are some common underlying problems that could be addressed by CDC and its partner institutions. These include a lack of awareness of the importance of these interventions among public health authorities, a lack of knowledge among the target populations, and economic and logistic barriers. In an effort to address these underlying problems, CDC and its public and private partner institutions have been bringing together experienced health communicators, economists, manufacturers, marketing experts, and other professionals with competencies not stressed by public health in the past. For example, through a partnership with Procter & Gamble, WHO, CARE, and USAID, CDC has made point-of-use chlorination of public drinking water available to about a million people in more than a dozen countries. This is a notable accomplishment; nonetheless, another estimated 1–1.5 billion people in the world still do not have safe drinking water and bear the brunt of diarrheal diseases and other waterborne infections as a result.

5. Global initiatives for disease control. CDC has been participating for many years in global initiatives for disease control, often in collaboration with WHO and other partners. Smallpox, polio, and dracunculiasis, for example, have been eradicated or are well on their way to being eradicated worldwide through partnerships that have included CDC. Other infectious diseases slated for eradication include measles, trachoma, and filariasis. These eradication campaigns are supported by dedicated staff in both Atlanta and the host countries, where CDC personnel advise national authorities on control strategies.

CDC has also dedicated significant human, financial, and scientific resources to many widely recognized global public health efforts, such as Roll Back Malaria, Stop TB, and the Global AIDS Program. The latter is one of the largest international programs in which CDC has ever been involved.

6. Public health training and capacity building. Although CDC has been involved in international public health training and capacity building for many years, its involvement in terms of financial resources has not been as great in this area as in some others. Nonetheless, there have been some significant successes, such as Field Epidemiology Training Programs and International Emerging Infectious Diseases Laboratory Fellowships. At the same time, significant benefits would accrue from additional investments in public health education and training on the part of CDC.

As with other priority areas in CDC's global infectious disease strategy, a heavy emphasis is placed on partnerships. CDC is actively working with The World Bank, USAID, the Rockefeller Foundation, the Lilly Foundation, and many others to develop training programs for epidemiologists and public health laboratory scientists. One of the new elements proposed in the CDC strategy is the creation of a series of International Emerging Infections Programs (IEIPs) that would serve as national and regional centers for surveillance, applied research, training, and education on diseases of national and global importance. The hope is that these new IEIPs will:

• Become the building blocks of a sophisticated international network that will conduct laboratory, population-based surveillance for a broad range of globally important infectious diseases.

• Be long-term, in-country partnerships and collaborations with ministry of health scientists that will be used to build an international and global capacity for disease control. Ministry of health and CDC scientists would train together while learning about the epidemiology and laboratory aspects of emerging infectious diseases.

• Provide a broad platform for basic and applied research on infectious diseases, including the development, application, implementation, and evaluation of public health tools.

•   Help support outbreak response efforts and, in so doing, strengthen the capacity to control emerging pathogens.

The first IEIP was launched in 2001 in Bangkok by the Thai Ministry of Health and Scott Dowell of CDC. The program works closely with the local Field Epidemiology Training Program and the local U.S. Department of Defense laboratory. At the time of the workshop, CDC hoped to choose the site for and launch the second IEIP later in 2002.

Response to the 2001 Anthrax Attacks: An Example of Effective Cooperation

Bioterrorism continues to shape and reshape both domestic and global public health agendas. Within hours of the first reports of bioterrorism-related anthrax in the United States, public health agencies around the world were faced with a myriad of questions from the highest levels of their governments, their clinicians and laboratory scientists, the media, and their citizens. Many of these agencies turned to CDC for information and advice. Over the period of a few short weeks, CDC received more than 160 calls and e-mails from officials and other individuals in about 70 countries requesting assistance or consultation on bioterrorism-related concerns. In many of these countries, the threat manifested itself as letters containing suspicious white powder that were delivered to various targets, including U.S. embassies, multinational corporate offices, local political groups, and ordinary citizens.

For example, the offices of a newspaper in Kurachi, Pakistan, were closed following the receipt of hate mail containing a suspicious white powder. A CDC colleague in a Karachi laboratory isolated gram-positive rods from the white powder and, suspecting that they were *Bacillus anthracis*, e-mailed a photograph of the bacteria to CDC in Atlanta. CDC microbiologists who were working with U.S. anthrax isolates were able to review the photo and provide direct consultation to individuals in Karachi. Later in the investigation, CDC arranged for the transfer of these isolates and highly suspect isolates from about a dozen other countries to the United States for testing by the U.S. Laboratory Response Network. Only three positive isolates were found—two in mail delivered to U.S. embassies in Peru and Vienna and the third in Chile.

Clearly, in this situation any government would be sensitive to information about anthrax-related bioterrorism or suspected bioterrorism in its own country. The willingness of so many ministries of health to collaborate closely with CDC and other U.S. institutions on these highly sensitive matters is a tribute to the trust and relationships that have developed in international public health over the years. More than 100 CDC employees assigned to countries worldwide received e-mail updates on the anthrax investigation and were able to serve as assistants or information sources for the local ministries of health, UN agencies, and U.S. embassies. The IEIP in Bangkok, Thailand, and the Southeast Asian regional office of WHO hosted a training course on anthrax during the investigation; there were more than 60 participants from 16 countries.

Partnering with the Developing World

Give a man a fish and you feed him for a day. Teach him how to fish and you feed him for a lifetime.

—Lao Tzu (Chinese Proverb)

Participants made several comments throughout the workshop regarding the manner in which the United States and other developed countries must interact with their partners in developing countries to ensure sustainable progress. Some of these comments were made within the context of opportunities for transnational research and training programs, such as the Gorgas Course (see Chapter 3); others were made within the context of the discussion on public–private partnerships summarized above.

First, past experience has shown that one of the critical prerequisites for a successful international health collaboration is for all involved to be treated as equal partners, especially when there are major disparities in resources. It is extremely important, whether the dialogue is about health or some other global issue, for developed countries to listen to their partners in developing countries and ask those involved to describe their problems and how interested developed countries can help resolve them.

The partnership between Instituto de Medicina Tropical "Alexander von Humboldt" in Lima, Peru, where the Gorgas Course is held, and the Belgian-run Institute of Tropical Medicine in Antwerp (described in Chapter 3) illustrate the value of this type of egalitarian approach. So, too, does the Southern Cone Initiative. Member countries were asked to list their top five problems, after which appropriate steps were taken, including the transfer of necessary technology and the implementation of training programs tailored to the needs and skill levels of the recipients. For example, Argentina listed hemolytic-uremic syndrome as one of its top public health problems; in response, steps were taken to provide the necessary resources, training, and technology transfer to help manage the problem.

Second, several participants expressed concern about the long-term sustainability of international collaborations. A foundation and methods need to be in place to sustain long-term collaborations among international partners in a mutually beneficial manner. The Fogarty International Center within NIH has taken a substantial step in the right direction by transitioning some of its collaborations to commitments of 10 years or longer. This should serve as a model for other coordination and partnership efforts (see Chapter 3 for additional details). In addition, CDC has indicated that it will be developing programs incorporating more permanent field involvement.

Third, the sharing of information between developed and developing countries should have practical benefit. Generally, collaborating countries expect to be informed of known best practices for addressing the specific problems they face. The mismanagement of dengue hemorrhagic fever by clinicians, for example, can have devastating consequences. Simple training, an understanding of the pathogenesis of the disease, and knowledge of the appropriate clinical interventions can dramatically reduce the mortality rate.

Fourth, when the United States implements initiatives or sends trainees or clinicians to the developing world, it is important for the experience to provide value to the host developing country. A participant questioned whether value is provided when trainees who may have idealistic notions about working in a developing country but are not even experienced enough to deal with patients in clinics in U.S. cities are sent to help those in need. A better approach might be to learn from the experiences and successes of local communities in resource-limited environments in the United States and then apply what has been learned in other settings.

Fifth, there is a critical need for bidirectionality in any international collaboration: developed and developing countries can learn equally from each other. The health of the populations and the economies of both can benefit. For example, many Latin American countries, as well as other countries worldwide, are learning important lessons about how to manage antimicrobial resistance; it would behoove all countries to learn these lessons. The same applies to food safety. As another example, clinicians in developed countries are ill prepared to address the multitude of infectious diseases that emerge among refugees or migrants from other parts of the world. Programs such as the Gorgas Course provide important training opportunities for clinicians from developed countries to see and observe first-hand diseases endemic to the developing world.

Finally, as history has shown, it is critical for local communities to be involved. For example, Peru has a long history of terrorism, perpetrated most notably by the Shining Path guerrillas (also known as Sendero Luminoso and the Communist Party of Peru). In the 1980s, the Shining Path was initially believed to be a small group distributed among very isolated villages. By the beginning of the 1990s, however, the group had claimed 20,000 lives and cost Peru an estimated $20 million. When the government, the police, intelligence officials, and especially the community at large realized the magnitude of the problem and made the decision to take control of the situation, the Shining Path leaders were captured within two months. One of the important lessons to be learned from Peru's experience with the Shining Path terrorists is that surveillance does not always reveal the magnitude of a problem and how that problem is developing. More important, Peru's experience illustrates the importance of different groups within a country working together and, in particular, of using the local community in combating a problem. This lesson has been learned repeatedly throughout history, from the U.S. experience in Vietnam to the costly experience with the 1991 South American cholera epidemic. With regard to the latter disease, in one Peruvian hospital today, for example, the rate of mortality from cholera is one per 2,000 cases, compared with one per 250 cases in the United States. This low mortality rate is due to a cooperative effort among scientists, academicians, politicians, public health workers, and the local community.

Infectious Disease Problems in the United States

Problems with emerging and reemerging infectious diseases are not confined to developing countries. As efforts to bridge the growing gap between the developed and developing worlds intensify, care must be taken not to lose sight of the serious infectious disease problems that exist in the United States and contribute to the global vulnerability to such diseases. There are many places in the United States where conditions are essentially the same as in developing countries. Several problems generally perceived to be problems of the developing world, such as improper adherence to medication regimens and limited access to health care, also occur in the United States. Indeed, some problems, such as multidrug resistance, are even worse in the United States and other developed nations than in the developing world.

Methicillin-resistant *Staphylococcus aureus* and ampicillin-resistant beta-lactamase-producing *Haemophilus influenzae* are two examples of drug-resistant microbes that are creating much greater public health problems in the United States than in most developing countries. Although the misuse of antibiotics is a major problem associated with the emergence of multidrug-resistant microbial strains, it was suggested that perhaps an even larger problem is person-to-person transmission of resistant strains, particularly in day-care centers, nursing homes, and hospitals. It was also noted that although antibiotic resistance occurs at a much lower rate in most developing countries than is currently the case in either the United States or Europe, there is good reason to expect that the world will soon have to deal with the problem on a much broader scale, including in developing countries. The issue of multidrug resistance was not discussed at length during the workshop, however; participants suggested that it should perhaps be reserved for in-depth discussion at another workshop.

Another issue of concern in the United States is how the new requirements for clinical trials will affect the development and Food and Drug Administration (FDA) approval of effective drugs. It was pointed out that the requirements are restricted to certain criteria; thus, they are not likely to be as detrimental as originally anticipated. That said, however, the requirement for larger numbers of patients for separate indications, even for the same antibiotic, in a clinical trial will clearly add to the cost of developing new antibiotics and, given competing costs and market opportunities, may discourage antibiotic research and development. FDA's Center for Drug Evaluation and Research is apparently addressing this issue and trying to distinguish requirements necessary to determine the appropriate use of antibiotics from those that would simply add expense to clinical trials.

THE NEED FOR A NEW, GLOBAL LEGAL FRAMEWORK[6]

The increasing global movement of people and products is forcing countries to confront heightened threats from the cross-border transmission of pathogenic microbes. Yet few if any domestic public health systems have adequate surveillance or other capabilities to manage these heightened threats independently. Public health capacity aside, unilateral efforts by individuals countries to manage public health threats that arise from cross-border microbial traffic can have only a limited impact when the source of the problem is beyond the jurisdiction and sovereignty of the affected country. Therefore, international law is a critical mechanism for facilitating an internationally cooperative public health response to the globalization of infectious disease.

Even before the current era of globalization and since the beginning of international cooperation on health-related matters in the mid-nineteenth century, international law has played an important role in facilitating intergovernmental cooperation in the control of infectious disease. The last several decades have, however, seen some significant shifts in this relationship between international law and infectious disease control. Never before has the role of international law been so important, or so uncertain. Although the IHRs have been revised to better accommodate the growing and urgent need for internationally coordinated response capabilities,[7] it is

---

[6]This section is based on the workshop presentations by Fidler (2002) and Klaucke (2002); see also Appendix B.

[7]Note that at the time of the workshop and the writing of this report, the IHRs had not yet been revised. The revised IHRs were adopted by the World Health Assembly on May 23, 2005.

unclear how the revised regulations will actually improve the ability to prevent and control infectious diseases.

The International Health Regulations: An Effort That Needs Improving

In 1995, the World Health Assembly voted to review and revise the IHRs. Their stated purpose, however, would remain the same: to "ensure the maximum security against the international spread of disease with a minimum interference with world traffic." The decision to revise the regulations was based on two major factors: (1) the public health need for more effective IHRs with respect to both emerging and reemerging infectious disease threats and vectors and the development of new technologies and approaches for controlling these diseases, and (2) environmental changes resulting from the globalization of markets, the increased transnational movement of goods and people, and the increased access to information.

Prior to being revised, IHRs specified that countries must notify WHO when cases of cholera, plague, and yellow fever arose and when areas were free of infection; required that ports, airports, and frontier posts be adequately equipped to apply the IHR measures; stated the maximum health measures applicable to international traffic, which a country could require for the protection of its territory against cholera, plague, and yellow fever; and required certain health documents, such as the Maritime Declaration of Health and Aircraft General Declaration. The IHRs were constrained in several ways: they were limited to three diseases; they depended on country notification to WHO; there was no mechanism for collaboration between individual countries and WHO; there was no incentive for countries to report; and they were limited in scope and lacked risk-specific measures for responding to urgent events.

The guiding principle of the revised IHRs is that the best way to prevent the international spread of disease is to detect public health threats early and to coordinate and implement an effective response when a problem is small and localized. Implementing this principle requires early detection of unusual disease events by an effective national disease surveillance system and an internationally coordinated response.

The revised IHRs have several important new features:

• They focus more on responding to unexpected events and improving preparedness at both the national and global levels. In contrast, the old IHRs were designed to contain known risks.
• They include procedures for real-time management in addition to the permanent procedures (e.g., environmental and epidemiological measures, such as insect and vector control) that were included in the old IHRs.

The information for real-time management is to be compiled from various IHR documents, such as regulations, annexes, and technical guides; the WHO-coordinated Global Outbreak Alert and Response Network (see the section on the use of the World Wide Web in international surveillance and response in Chapter 3); WHO-based epidemic intelligence; and IHR focal points in every country. A key component of the real-time event management aspect of the revised IHRs is confidential, or provisional, notification. Countries can enter into a dialogue with WHO regarding the best way to control a situation without the dialogue becoming general knowledge. Other real-time management features of the revised IHRs include WHO's ability to accept information from unofficial sources, after which verification would be obtained from the country; WHO's provision of network response support; and the availability of a template of recommendations and measures based on risk assessments for particular events.

• Under the new IHRs, each country is required to maintain core surveillance capacities, as defined in the IHRs, including the ability to detect and report infectious diseases and to respond at both the local public health and national levels. Initially, this will be a target capacity for many countries, and WHO will need to work with these countries to develop their capacities. Each country will receive technical guidelines for the establishment of early-warning systems.

• The criteria for reporting under the new IHRs include "public health emergencies of international concern." WHO and the Swedish Institute of Infectious Diseases have been developing an algorithm for determining when a public health emergency may have an international effect and thus whether WHO should be notified. Following notification of WHO, consultation and collaboration between the country and WHO will be used to determine the appropriate response. The four main components of the algorithm are as follows: Is this event serious? Is it unexpected? Could it or has it spread internationally? Is there a risk of international sanctions?

Of course, even the revised IHRs will face numerous challenges:

• Convincing countries that notification of urgent public events under the new IHRs is to their advantage.

• Ensuring that international reactions to events are appropriate and that other countries do not impose inappropriate sanctions.

• Developing the national political will to detect, investigate, and control problems instead of ignoring them and waiting for them to disappear (which has often been the case in the past for those diseases not required to be reported).

• Developing the national capacity for surveillance and response.

International Law and Emerging Infectious Diseases

The public health challenges created by globalization can be categorized conceptually as either vertical or horizontal. Vertical challenges represent problems countries face within their own borders, such as weak surveillance capabilities. Horizontal challenges are the public health problems that arise from increased cross-border traffic of microbes resulting from the greater speed and volume of international trade and travel. Public health strategies against infectious diseases can be similarly categorized. A vertical strategy is an attempt to reduce the prevalence of an infectious disease inside a single country from within that country. In contrast, a horizontal strategy is an attempt to create cooperation among countries to minimize disease exportation and importation.

Usually, the onus of implementing both types of strategies falls on the individual country. After all, public health is a public good, which means it is the government's responsibility; private-sector actors have neither the resources nor the incentives to do what is necessary to protect the public's health. Thus, the individual country is a critical component of the governance response to emerging and reemerging infectious disease threats. It can operate within one of three overlapping governance frameworks:

- A national governance response occurs within a country's territory and under its own laws, and as such is a vertical strategy. For example, national quarantine practices in the first half of the nineteenth century took place without international cooperation; each country managed its own strategy with regard to infectious disease threats.
- An international governance response is the classic intergovernmental cooperation that occurs, for example, in WHO or the World Trade Organization (WTO). International governance is aimed primarily at creating horizontal public health strategies regarding disease exportation and importation. The IHRs are an example of such a response.
- A global governance response involves nonstate actors—including multinational corporations and NGOs—all of which play a significant and sometimes formal role in handling issues at the global level. At this level, the multinational corporations and NGOs are effectively built into the governmental response mechanisms. The primary strategic emphasis of global governance is vertical. The attempt is to reach down to the local level, and there is little interest in intergovernmental cooperation. The role of international law in global governance is not structural; rather, it is to provide norms that influence vertical public health strategies. The Global Fund is an example of global governance.

The first century of international health diplomacy, which began in the mid-1800s, witnessed the creation of three primary horizontal international legal regimes relating to infectious diseases: the classical, organizational, and trade regimes. The classical regime dates back to the inception of the early International Sanitary Convention in 1851, which was replaced by the International Sanitary Regulations in 1951 and then renamed the IHRs in 1969. The IHRs' stated purpose—"to ensure the maximum protection against the international spread of disease with minimum interference with world traffic"—captures the essence of the classical regime, which constitutes the central and most important use of international law in infectious disease governance at the international level, at least within the first 100 years of international health diplomacy.

The organizational regime represents the various state-created international health organizations (IHOs), beginning in 1902 with the Pan American Sanitary Bureau. This regime involves the use of international law to create permanent IHOs, such as today's WHO, in an effort to facilitate intergovernmental cooperation on infectious diseases and other international public health problems. In contrast with the classical regime, the organizational regime's legal responsibilities for infectious disease control have been shallow at best.

The best example of the trade regime, which represents efforts to liberalize trade among states, is the General Agreement on Tariffs and Trade (GATT), adopted in 1947. Although its explicit purpose is not infectious disease control, GATT includes rules that allow states to restrict trade to protect human, plant, and animal life and health. Thus, it figures in the use of international law in the international governance of infectious disease control.

Over the last five decades, there have been several important shifts in governance with important implications for infectious disease control. First, within the realm of horizontal international governance, there has been a shift in emphasis from the classical to the trade regime. This was evident in the number of times WTO was mentioned during the workshop and is referred to in this report—far more times than either the IHRs, which represent the classical regime, or WHO, which represents the organizational regime. The classical regime has been widely recognized as failing to achieve its objective of maximum protection against the international spread of disease with minimum interference with world traffic, for several reasons (see the preceding section on the IHRs). WTO came into existence in 1995, almost simultaneously with WHO's recognition that the IHRs were inadequate to deal with the challenges posed by globalization.

Since its inception, WTO has become the central horizontal regime for international law on infectious diseases. Two WTO agreements in particular have garnered attention: the Agreement on Trade-Related Aspects of Intellectual Property Rights (the TRIPS agreement) and the Agreement on the Application of Sanitary and Phytosanitary Measures (SPS Agreement) in connection with food safety.

This shift from the classical to the trade regime raises some questions with regard to WHO's revision of the IHRs. Participants suggested that there was some indication that a revised set of IHRs might not even be necessary. For example, with regard to maximum protection against the spread of infectious disease, there has been a shift away from relying on the binding legal duty to provide notification of specific diseases to a reliance in WHO on new information technologies. This shift is epitomized by WHO's Global Outbreak Alert and Response Network, which is being used to gather global epidemiological information outside the framework of the IHRs. It is unclear whether the IHRs are necessary for WHO to make progress on global epidemiological surveillance. As another example and with regard to minimum interference with traffic and trade, many irrational trade-restricting health measures are sometimes instituted when countries report real or supposed disease outbreaks (see Chapter 3). Despite WHO's attempt to give the IHRs more teeth to deal with the issue, WHO is no longer the most important player, but WTO. Not only does this shift from the classical to the trade regime raise questions about the usefulness of the IHRs and the need to develop revised IHRs, but it also raises the question of whether we are witnessing the rejuvenation of the classical regime or its death.

A second change that has occurred over the past several decades with regard to the governance of infectious diseases is the evolution after World War II of vertical international regimes that influence global strategies on infectious disease much more dramatically than do the traditional horizontal approaches. Although these regimes—the soft-law regime, the environmental regime, and the human rights regime—are not international, their objectives are to deal with issues that concern individual countries and to improve conditions inside countries; their purpose is not necessarily to regulate intergovernmental cooperation.

For example, the soft-law regime, which includes WHO's development of norms, principles, guidelines, and best practices on infectious disease control (e.g., the DOTS strategy for TB control), is not legally binding on WHO member states (hence the term "soft law"). Indeed, voluntary compliance is an important aspect of how WHO has historically worked. Adoption of these norms and practices generally has a beneficial impact inside the country for both the government and the public health system. Unfortunately, compliance with soft-law guidance from WHO is not very good, as the lack of compliance with DOTS illustrates.

The environmental regime, another development after World War II, is an attempt to improve environmental practices inside countries so that their populations can enjoy better environmental conditions. Thus, to many people's surprise, it is also an international body of law concerned with the protection of human health. One of its weaknesses with respect to infectious disease, however, is that it focuses very little if at all on local air and water pollution, two of the greatest environmental sources of morbidity and mortality from infectious disease.

The human rights regime, which imposes obligations on governments in connection with their treatment of persons living within their territories, also has the potential to have a significant effect on public health. Respect for human rights, including the right to health, has been part of strategies for dealing with a number of public health crises, including the HIV/AIDS pandemic, as well as treaties such as the UN Convention on the Rights of the Child. This regime is now quite powerful.

A third critical change in governance of infectious disease over the last 50 years is the development of global governance mechanisms that support the new trade and vertical public health strategies. Again, unlike international governance, which involves only states, global governance involves states, intergovernmental organizations, and nonstate actors, and the strategy is vertical, not horizontal. The involvement of NGOs and multinational corporations is a key component of these new mechanisms, whose strategic objective is to produce global public goods that states, especially developing countries, can use within their own territories to reduce the rates of morbidity and mortality from infectious disease. Currently, one of the most prominent features of these new global governance mechanisms is the development of public–private partnerships, such as the Global Fund. As another example, infectious disease surveillance, especially via the Global Outbreak and Alert Response Network (see Chapter 3), is often fueled by the participation of nongovernmental actors who acquire their information from nongovernmental sources, such as the press, the online website ProMED, and NGOs.

One of the most controversial developments in the infectious disease arena as regards global governance is the development of the new access regime, which arose from a clash between the trade and human rights regimes. The objective of the access regime is to improve access to essential drugs, vaccines, and medicines in developing countries; the regime is being driven largely by nonstate actors, as opposed to intergovernmental organizations or states, and is characterized by the heavy involvement of NGOs (e.g., the Global Fund and the Global Alliance for Vaccines and Immunization). The emergence of the access regime was marked by the dramatic adoption of the Declaration on the TRIPS Agreement and Public Health at the WTO Doha Ministerial Meeting in November 2001. The declaration clearly supports placing public health objectives, especially access to medicines, above the trade-related goal of increasing patent protection for pharmaceuticals. Experts view the declaration as a victory for the human right to health and for public health governance generally.

Another development involves arguments that infectious diseases represent national security threats, and as such should be a priority on foreign policy agendas. In contrast to the movement toward vertical global governance characteristic of the access regime, these arguments seek to reconnect infectious disease control with national and international governance by reengaging the great powers in international public health. Should these arguments take hold, one might foresee reinvigorated national and international governance on infectious disease.

However, it would be prudent to be cautious about arguments that infectious diseases represent national security and foreign policy threats. Historically, the great powers have not hesitated to bend, break, or abandon international law when they believed national security was being threatened. Although the United States has focused energy and new funding on homeland security against bioterrorism, it has rejected multilateral efforts to strengthen international governance as it pertains to the threat of biological weapons. Many experts are concerned about what appears to be a rejuvenated U.S. unilateralism in an area in which public health plays a strategic role.

At the same time, the tepid and tardy responses to the HIV/AIDS catastrophe in sub-Saharan Africa hardly suggest that infectious disease problems in faraway countries have risen high on many national security and foreign policy agendas. The shift from binding commitments in international governance efforts to nonbinding, voluntary participation in global governance efforts may suit the narrow public health interests of the great powers at the expense of strengthening national and international governance of infectious disease.

Never before has the role of international law been so important in infectious disease control. At the same time, there is a great deal of uncertainty about where these new developments will lead and whether they will really have an impact on improving the ability to prevent and control infectious disease at the global level.

THE NEED FOR A SOCIAL SCIENTIFIC FRAMEWORK FOR UNDERSTANDING INFECTIOUS DISEASE EMERGENCE[8]

Attempts to understand the etiology of the emergence of infectious diseases cannot be restricted to a purely biological approach. Rarely, if ever, is the emergence of an infectious disease caused exclusively by biological factors. The word "syndemic" was recently introduced into the English language to refer to the convergence of factors that typically contribute to

---

[8]This section is based on the workshop presentations by Mayer (2002) and Patz (2002); see also Appendix C.

the emergence of infectious diseases (Singer, 1994). This is perhaps no better illustrated than by the emergence of West Nile virus in New York City, an event that was the culmination of the convergence of a number of different human ecological factors.

Only by studying the complex interplay among the social, environmental, and biological factors that underlie the emergence of infectious disease can one hope to gain an understanding of disease distribution patterns and changes. In the original IOM (1992) report on microbial threats, *Emerging Infections: Microbial Threats to Human Health in the United States*, five of the six factors identified as contributing to the emergence of infectious disease are explicitly social in nature (i.e., human demographics and behavior, technology and industry, economic development and land use, international travel and commerce, and a breakdown in public health), and the sixth (microbial adaptation and change) is partly the result of social behavior and social change.[9] The effects of dam construction, land clearance projects, and other environmental modifications on vector ecology illustrate the necessity of adopting a social approach to understanding the global emergence of infectious diseases. To understand the effects of globalization on vector ecology, one must study not only vector ecologies per se, but also the role of human activities and behaviors.

Despite the vital role of social factors in the etiology of infectious disease emergence and the fact that the literatures of many of the social sciences, such as demography and political geography, could inform our understanding of infectious disease emergence, the vast preponderance of research and policy on the emergence of infectious diseases has been explicitly biological in nature. Little social science has been incorporated into epidemiological, public health, or infectious disease research and policy.

One of the consequences of the failure to take a social scientific perspective in attempting to understand the emergence of infectious diseases has been a restrictive definition of globalization in public health—a definition that tends to focus only on surface phenomena, such as the movement of people and commodities. Even within the workshop, as summarized in Chapter 1, most of the descriptions of phenomena that characterize the globalization of infectious disease revolved around the movement and interaction of people and goods. There was comparatively little discussion on the movement of capital and the critical role of political and economic

---

[9]In the IOM (2003) report that was the successor to the 1992 report, *Microbial Threats to Health: Emergence, Detection, and Response*, 10 of the 13 identified factors in emergence are explicitly social in nature; the other three (microbial adaptation and change, climate and weather, and changing ecosystems) are at least partly the result of social behavior and social change.

decision-making power that transcends national borders. Yet understanding the relationships between changing vector ecologies, for example, and globalization necessitates an understanding of how political and economic decisions, particularly those that alter the landscape, change human–environment relations at the local, regional, and global levels. Failure to recognize the importance of the latter could compromise efforts to strengthen the global capacity to prevent and control emerging and re-emerging infectious diseases.

How can a social scientific perspective be incorporated into the study of emerging and reemerging infectious diseases? Classic geographic disease ecology has been developing since about the time of World War II, when Jacques May, a French surgeon who practiced in French Indochina, became intrigued by the role of the interaction of local social, cultural, and environmental conditions in the development of patterns of contagion for a number of infectious diseases. He eventually gave up his surgical career to become the medical geographer at the American Geographical Society in New York City, where he produced numerous volumes and papers on disease ecology, including a monumental 30-volume collection of works demonstrating how disease ecology could be understood from a more integrated and less purely biological perspective (May, 1958). As significant as his work was, however, May did not consider the impact of other regions on local conditions. Thus, even though interregional patterns of commodity shipments, cultural contact, and cultural change are aspects of global interdependency that were apparent decades ago, May did not incorporate them in his descriptions and analyses. Nor did he consider the effects of power and politics on local disease conditions. That tradition has continued to today. Even when social factors are considered, disease ecologists tend to focus only on isolated regions and generally fail to consider regional hierarchies and interregional interactions and flows, such as the migration of people and the movement of capital.

The political ecology of disease may provide the best way yet to conceptualize the impact of these factors on local disease ecologies. Political ecology, which is based on a combination of political economy and cultural ecology, is "the attempt to understand the political sources, conditions, and ramifications of environmental change" (Bryant, 1992, p. 13). It can and has been used as a way to understand the unintended consequences of environmental decisions, particularly those, such as dam building, that alter human–environment relations and affect emerging infectious diseases (Mayer, 2000).

In addition to adopting a political ecology approach, another means suggested for improving the conceptual framework for understanding the emergence of infectious diseases is to strengthen the type of interdisciplinary research that addresses key knowledge gaps related to how factors of emergence converge and interact. This will be a challenging task, as it will require long-term cross-disciplinary collaboration. As an example of the current failure of cross-disciplinary communication, not a single climatologist was included in a recent multiauthored paper on climate and malaria in the African Highlands published in the journal *Nature*, even though the work was essentially a climate study and made use of an extant climate database (Hay et al., 2002). Indeed, the climatologist whose climate database was used in the study prepared a rebuttal for publication in the journal pointing out how the database was used inappropriately and how the results are flawed. If a climatologist had been part of the original research team, this situation could have been avoided.

As the impacts of dam construction and land modification projects on emerging infectious diseases attest (see Chapter 1), the need to understand emergence within the larger social and political context is clearly not just an academic exercise. Human activity associated with the expansion of free-market capitalism threatens to destroy ecosystems and opens the door to the rapid emergence of new diseases. If left unchecked, the current economic model that allows such environmental devastation will likely lead to future public health crises. Moreover, recent research suggests that scarcities of vital environmental resources—especially cropland, freshwater, and forests—contribute to violence in many parts of the world, a phenomenon that feeds back into and amplifies the effect of the devastation. As the competition for scarce resources increases, environmental devastation worsens, the potential for economic prosperity decreases, and public health deteriorates.

REFERENCES

Adeyi O. 2002 (April 17). *Considerations for Shaping the Agenda*. Presentation at the Institute of Medicine Workshop on the Impact of Globalization on Infectious Disease Emergence and Control: Exploring the Consequences and Opportunities, Washington, D.C. Institute of Medicine Forum on Emerging Infections.

Bryant RL. 1992. Political ecology: An emerging research agenda in third world studies. *Political Geography* 11(1):12–36.

Cash R. 2002 (April 16). *Impediments to Global Surveillance and Open Reporting of Infectious Diseases*. Presentation at the Institute of Medicine Workshop on the Impact of Globalization on Infectious Disease Emergence and Control: Exploring the Consequences and Opportunities, Washington, D.C. Institute of Medicine Forum on Emerging Infections.

CDC (Centers for Disease Control and Prevention). 2002. *Protecting the Nation's Health in an Era of Globalization: CDC's Global Infectious Disease Strategy*. Atlanta, GA. [Online]. Available: http://www.cdc.gov/globalidplan/global_id_plan.pdf [accessed September 12, 2005].

Cleghorn F. 2002 (April 16). *Considering the Resources and the Capacity for the Response*. Presentation at the Institute of Medicine Workshop on the Impact of Globalization on Infectious Disease Emergence and Control: Exploring the Consequences and Opportunities, Washington, D.C. Institute of Medicine Forum on Emerging Infections.

Fidler D. 2002 (April 16). *International Law, Infectious Disease, and Globalization*. Presentation at the Institute of Medicine Workshop on the Impact of Globalization on Infectious Disease Emergence and Control: Exploring the Consequences and Opportunities, Washington, D.C. Institute of Medicine Forum on Emerging Infections.

Gardner P. 2002 (April 17). *New Directions in Capacity Building*. Presentation at the Institute of Medicine Workshop on the Impact of Globalization on Infectious Disease Emergence and Control: Exploring the Consequences and Opportunities, Washington, D.C. Institute of Medicine Forum on Emerging Infections.

Gordon D. 2002 (April 16). *The Global Infectious Disease Threat*. Presentation at the Institute of Medicine Workshop on the Impact of Globalization on Infectious Disease Emergence and Control: Exploring the Consequences and Opportunities, Washington, D.C. Institute of Medicine Forum on Emerging Infections.

Hay SI, Cox J, Rogers DJ, Randolph SE, Stern DI, Shanks GD, Myers MF, Snow RW. 2002. Climate change and the resurgence of malaria in the East African Highlands. *Nature* 415(6874):905–909.

IOM (Institute of Medicine). 1992. *Emerging Infections: Microbial Threats to Health in the United States*. Washington, D.C.: National Academy Press.

IOM. 2003. *Microbial Threats to Health: Emergence, Detection, and Response*. Washington, D.C.: The National Academies Press.

Kimball AM. 2002 (April 16). *Invited Discussion: Considering the Resources and Capacity for the Response*. Presentation at the Institute of Medicine Workshop on the Impact of Globalization on Infectious Disease Emergence and Control: Exploring the Consequences and Opportunities, Washington, D.C. Institute of Medicine Forum on Emerging Infections.

Klaucke D. 2002. *Globalization and Health: A Framework for Analysis and Action*. Presentation at the Institute of Medicine Workshop on the Impact of Globalization on Infectious Disease Emergence and Control: Exploring the Consequences and Opportunities, Washington, D.C. Institute of Medicine Forum on Emerging Infections.

Kurth R. 2002 (April 17). *The Global Application of Tools, Technology, and Knowledge to Counter the Consequences of Infectious Diseases: A Discussion of Priorities and Options*. Presentation at the Institute of Medicine Workshop on the Impact of Globalization on Infectious Disease Emergence and Control: Exploring the Consequences and Opportunities, Washington, D.C. Institute of Medicine Forum on Emerging Infections.

Leaning J. 2002 (April 16). *Health, Human Rights, and Humanitarian Assistance: The Medical and Public Health Response to Crises and Disasters*. Presentation at the Institute of Medicine Workshop on the Impact of Globalization on Infectious Disease Emergence and Control: Exploring the Consequences and Opportunities, Washington, D.C. Institute of Medicine Forum on Emerging Infections.

LeDuc J. 2002 (April 17). *The Global Application of Tools, Technology, and Knowledge to Counter the Consequences of Infectious Diseases: A Discussion of Priorities and Options*. Presentation at the Institute of Medicine Workshop on the Impact of Globalization on Infectious Disease Emergence and Control: Exploring the Consequences and Opportunities, Washington, D.C. Institute of Medicine Forum on Emerging Infections.

May JM. 1958. *The Ecology of Human Disease*. New York: M.D. Publications.

Mayer JD. 2000. Geography, ecology, and emerging infectious diseases. *Social Science and Medicine* 50(7-8):937–952.

Mayer JD. 2002 (April 16). *The Global Movement of Populations, Products, and Pathogens*. Presentation at the Institute of Medicine Workshop on the Impact of Globalization on Infectious Disease Emergence and Control: Exploring the Consequences and Opportunities, Washington, D.C. Institute of Medicine Forum on Emerging Infections.

NIC (National Intelligence Council). 2000. National intelligence estimate: The global infectious disease threat and its implications for the United States. *Environ Change Secur Proj Rep* 2(6):33–65.

Patz J. 2002 (April 16). *Invited Discussion: Considering the Resources and Capacity for the Response*. Presentation at the Institute of Medicine Workshop on the Impact of Globalization on Infectious Disease Emergence and Control: Exploring the Consequences and Opportunities, Washington, D.C. Institute of Medicine Forum on Emerging Infections.

Singer M. 1994. AIDS and the health crisis of the U.S. urban poor: The perspective of critical medical anthropology. *Social Science and Medicine* 39(7):931–948.

Steiger W. 2002 (April 17). *The Global Fund: A Brave New World*. Presentation at the Institute of Medicine Workshop on the Impact of Globalization on Infectious Disease Emergence and Control: Exploring the Consequences and Opportunities, Washington, D.C. Institute of Medicine Forum on Emerging Infections.

WHO (World Health Organization). 2000 (April). *Economic Costs of Malaria Are Many Times Higher Than Previously Estimated*. Press Release WHO/28, 25. Joint report issued by the World Health Organization, Harvard University, and the London School of Hygiene and Tropical Medicine at the African Summit on Roll Back Malaria in Abuja, Nigeria. [Online]. Available: http://www.who.int/inf-pr-2000/en/pr2000-28.html [accessed September 12, 2005].

Widdus R. 2002 (April 17). *Partnering for Success: The Role of Private-Public Sector Collaboration*. Presentation at the Institute of Medicine Workshop on the Impact of Globalization on Infectious Disease Emergence and Control: Exploring the Consequences and Opportunities, Washington, D.C. Institute of Medicine Forum on Emerging Infections.

World Bank. 2000. *Economic Analysis of HIV/AIDS. ADF 2000 Background Paper*. AIDS Campaign Team for Africa. Washington, D.C.: The World Bank.

Appendix A

Agenda

FORUM ON EMERGING INFECTIONS

Board on Global Health
Institute of Medicine
The National Academies

THE IMPACT OF GLOBALIZATION ON INFECTIOUS
DISEASE EMERGENCE AND CONTROL:
EXPLORING THE CONSEQUENCES AND OPPORTUNITIES

April 16–17, 2002

AGENDA

Tuesday, April 16, 2002

8:30   Continental Breakfast

9:00   **Welcome and Opening Remarks**
        Adel Mahmoud, President, Merck Vaccines
        Chair
        Forum on Emerging Infections

Session I: The Global Movement of Populations, Products, and Pathogens

Moderator: James Hughes, Assistant Surgeon General and Director,
National Center for Infectious Diseases, CDC

9:15   **The World and Its Moving Parts**
        Martin Cetron, Deputy Director, Division of Quarantine,
        National Center for Infectious Diseases, CDC

9:35   Global Migration and Infectious Diseases
        Danielle Grondin, Director, Migration Health Services,
        International Organization of Migration

9:55   Globalization of the Food Supply
        David Acheson, Chief Medical Officer, Food Safety and
        Inspection Service, USDA

10:15   Changing Vector Ecologies: Political Geographic
        Perspectives
        Jonathan Mayer, Professor, Geography, College of Arts and
        Sciences, University of Washington, Seattle

10:35   BREAK

10:50   Invited Discussion: A Response to the Shifting Trends

        Moderator: Margaret Hamburg, Vice-President, Biologicals
        Program, Nuclear Threat Initiative
        Stephen Corber, Director, Division of Disease Prevention
        and Control, Pan American Health Organization
        Mary Wilson, Professor of Medicine, Harvard Medical
        School, Population and International Health
        Judith Miller, Journalist, the *New York Times*
        David Heyman, Senior Fellow, Center for Strategic and
        International Studies

12:30   Lunch

   Session II: Addressing the Health Challenges from Globalization

Moderator: Patrick Kelley, Director, DoD Global Emerging Infections
Surveillance and Response Systems, Walter Reed Army Institute of
Research

1:30   The Global Infectious Disease Threat
        David Gordon, Intelligence Officer, Economics and Global
        Health Issues, National Intelligence Council

1:50   Health, Human Rights, and Humanitarian Assistance: The
        Medical and Public Health Response to Crises and Disasters
        Jennifer Leaning, Professor, Population and International
        Health, Harvard University

2:10   **Social Aspects of Public Health Challenges in a Period of Globalization: The Case of Russia**
Andrey Demin, President, Russian Public Health Association and Professor, I.M. Sechenov Medical Academy, Moscow

2:30   **Considerations for Drug Access and Delivery in the Developing World**
Robert Redfield, Professor and Associate Director, Institute of Human Virology, University of Maryland, Baltimore

2:50   **Impediments to Global Surveillance and Open Reporting of Infectious Diseases**
Richard Cash, Lecturer on International Health, Harvard School of Public Health

3:10   **International Law, Infectious Disease, and Globalization**
David Fidler, Professor of Law and Ira C. Batman Faculty Fellow, School of Law, Indiana University

3:30   BREAK

3:45   **Invited Discussion: Considering the Resources and Capacity for the Response**

        Moderator: Stanley Lemon, Dean of Medicine, University of Texas, Medical Branch, Galveston
Farley Cleghorn, Senior Scientist, Institute of Human Virology, University of Maryland, Baltimore
Ann Marie Kimball, Professor, Epidemiology and Health Services, University of Washington, Seattle
Michele Barry, President, American Society of Tropical Medicine and Hygiene, Professor, Yale University, School of Medicine
Jonathan Patz, Associate Professor, Bloomberg School of Public Health, Johns Hopkins University

5:30   **Adjournment of the first day**

5:45   **Reception, Members Room of the NAS**

6:15   **Dinner Meeting for Forum Members**

Wednesday, April 17, 2002

8:30   Continental Breakfast

9:00   Opening Remarks/Day One Summary
         Stanley Lemon
         Vice-Chair, Forum on Emerging Infections

Session III: Creating Opportunities from Globalization: A Framework for Progress

Moderator: Michael Zeilinger, Public Health Advisor, Team Leader, Infectious Diseases, USAID

9:15   Globalization and Health: A Framework for Analysis and
         Action
         Douglas Klaucke, Communicable Disease Surveillance and
         Response, World Health Organization

9:35   New Directions in Capacity Building
         Pierce Gardner, Senior Advisor for Clinical Research and
         Training, Fogarty International Center, NIH

9:55   Partnering for Success: The Role of Private-Public Sector
         Collaboration
         Roy Widdus, Project Manager, Initiative for Public-Private
         Partnerships for Health, Geneva

10:15   The Current Situation and Perspectives of International
         Collaboration in the Field of Biomedical Sciences: The
         Example of the State Research Center of Virology and
         Biotechnology (VECTOR)
         Sergei Netesov, Deputy Director, VECTOR Laboratories,
         Koltsovo, Russia

10:35   Protecting the Nation's Health in an Era of Globalization,
         CDC's Global Infectious Disease Strategy
         Eric Mintz, Acting Associate Director for Global Health, CDC

10:55   The Global Fund: A Brave New World
         William Steiger, Special Assistant to the Secretary,
         International Affairs, Department of Health and Human
         Services

11:15   BREAK

11:30   Invited Discussion: Considerations for Shaping the Agenda

Moderator: Carlos Lopez, Research Fellow, Eli Lilly and Company

> Olusoj Adeyi, Senior Health Specialist, World Bank
> William Makgoba, President, Medical Research Council of
> South Africa *(by teleconference)*
> Mark Miller, Associate Director for Research and Director,
> Division of International Epidemiology and Population
> Studies, Fogarty International Center, NIH
> Ralph Timperi, Chair, APHL Global Health Committee and
> Assistant Commissioner/Director, State Laboratory Institute
> Massachusetts Department of Public Health

1:00   **Lunch**

**Session IV: The Global Application of Tools, Technology, and
Knowledge to Counter the Consequences of Infectious Diseases:
A Discussion of Priorities and Options**

2:00   With the backdrop of the two days' presentations and
discussion, Forum members, panel discussants, and the
audience will comment on the issues and next steps that they
would identify as priority areas for consideration within
industry, academia, government agencies, public health
organizations, and other nongovernmental organizations. The
discussion of priorities will summarize the issues surrounding
emerging opportunities for more effective collaboration as well
as the options and considerations for research, development,
and capacity building. The complexities of interaction among
private industry, research and public health agencies,
regulatory agencies, policymakers, academic researchers, and
the public will be explored with an eye toward innovative
responses to the challenges and opportunities presented by an
increasingly "globalized" world.

Moderator: Adel Mahmoud, President, Merck Vaccines

Invited Panel Discussants:
Eduardo Gotuzzo, President, Latin American Society of
Tropical Medicine and Principal Professor, University Perudad
Cayetano Heredia, Peru
Reinhard Kurth, President, the Robert Koch Institute, Berlin
Jim LeDuc, Acting Director, Division of Viral and Rickettsial
Diseases, Centers for Disease Control and Prevention

3:30   **Roundtable Discussion**

4:30   **Closing Remarks / Adjournment**
Adel Mahmoud, President, Merck Vaccines
Chair, Forum on Emerging Infections

Appendix B

International Law, Infectious Diseases, and Globalization[1]

David P. Fidler[2]

P ublic health experts recognize that globalization creates challenges for infectious disease policy nationally and internationally. These challenges are many and diverse, but conceptually, they can be categorized as *horizontal* and *vertical* health challenges. Horizontal challenges constitute the public health problems that arise from increased cross-border microbial traffic caused by the increased speed and volume of international trade and travel. The global movement of populations and products forces countries to confront heightened threats from the cross-border transmission of pathogenic microbes. The horizontal challenges are, thus, policy challenges among many states.

Increased cross-border microbial traffic through globalization reveals weaknesses in domestic public health systems, such as inadequate surveillance capabilities. The vertical challenges represent the problems that countries face inside their territories, from the national to the local level. Responses to vertical challenges aim, therefore, to reform public health practices and policies within a state but not between states.

Experience with the effect of globalization on infectious disease control and prevention demonstrates that states cannot deal with the horizontal or vertical challenges adequately without cooperation. Unilateral state efforts against cross-border pathogen traffic can have only limited impact when

[1]Portions of this appendix are based on Fidler (2001a).
[2]Professor of Law and Ira C. Batman Faculty Fellow, Indiana University School of Law, 211 South Indiana Avenue, Bloomington, IN 47405, dfidler@indiana.edu.

the source of the problem is beyond the jurisdiction and sovereignty of the state affected. Similarly, many countries, especially developing countries, need assistance from other states and international organizations in order to improve domestic public health. Mechanisms to facilitate international cooperation, such as international law, are crucial to public health responses to the consequences of globalization for infectious disease prevention and control.

This appendix examines how international law relates to the horizontal and vertical challenges for infectious disease policy created by globalization. International law forms part of governance response to globalization, which is explored in the first section. The second section looks at the development of horizontal international legal regimes relating to infectious diseases that developed in the first century of international health diplomacy, 1851–1951. The last 50 years have, however, witnessed changes in how international law relates to the governance challenges globalization creates for infectious disease policy; these changes are analyzed in the third section. The final section examines how current arguments connecting infectious diseases with foreign policy and national security concerns of the great powers might affect the role of international law in global infectious disease policy.

GOVERNANCE RESPONSES TO THE CHALLENGES OF GLOBALIZATION

Vertical and Horizontal Strategies for Infectious Disease Control

The challenges globalization presents for infectious disease policy demand governance responses. For the horizontal challenges posed by cross-border microbial traffic, the governance response centers on building interstate cooperation to minimize disease exportation and importation (see Figure B-1). The vertical challenges of inadequate public health systems inside states require strategies that seek to reduce the infectious disease prevalence within states through improvement of domestic public health performance (see Figure B-2). The construction of vertical and horizontal strategies on infectious diseases constitutes the fundamental objective of public health governance in the era of globalization, but as detailed in the next subsection, governance responses to globalization challenges come in three primary forms that ultimately are interdependent.

Three Governance Frameworks

The state and its government constitute the key actor in public health governance for infectious diseases. Public health is a "public good," the

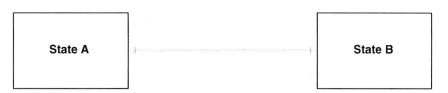

Horizontal Strategy: Cooperation
between states A and B to minimize
infectious disease exportation and
importation

FIGURE B-1   Horizontal strategies for infectious disease control.

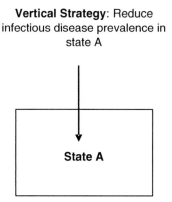

FIGURE B-2   Vertical strategies for infectious disease control.

production of which falls to the public sector because private actors lack sufficient incentives or resources to do what is necessary to protect population health (Gostin, 2001). When globalization pressures a state, its governance response can occur within three different governance categories: national, international, and global (see Figure B-3).

National governance represents the efforts a state takes within its own territory and under its own laws to respond to globalization-related problems. *International governance* means that states engage in international cooperation among themselves to confront globalization challenges. International governance often involves the creation of norms, rules, and institutions to facilitate interstate cooperation. The policies and duties created through international governance then inform national governance. *Global governance* involves not only states and international institutions but also nonstate actors, such as multinational corporations (MNCs) and international non-

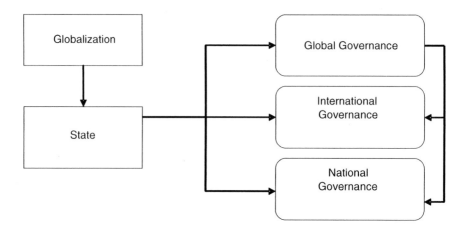

FIGURE B-3   Governance responses to globalization challenges.

governmental organizations (NGOs) (Dodgson et al., 2002). MNCs and NGOs shoulder governance roles because their participation and input become critical to the success of the overall endeavor. Global governance efforts affect the dynamics of both international and national governance.

International Law, Infectious Disease Strategies, and the Governance Frameworks

Crudely defined, international law constitutes the body of binding rules that govern the relations between sovereign states (Brownlie, 1998). Rules of international law apply to nonstate actors, as the body of international human rights law demonstrates, but the bulk of contemporary international law still regulates the intercourse between sovereign states. International law exhibits different functions within the contexts of both vertical and horizontal public health strategies on infectious diseases and the three governance frameworks. Table B-1 summarizes the various functions of international law in these two contexts.

The different strategic emphases in the three governance frameworks and the differing functions of international law exhibited in Table B-1 can be delineated through a historical overview of the development of governance on infectious diseases in response to globalization challenges. The next two sections provide this historical analysis.

TABLE B-1   Governance Frameworks, Public Health Strategies, and
International Law on Infectious Diseases

Governance Framework	Primary Strategic Emphasis	Function of International Law	Infectious Disease Example
National Governance	Vertical strategies	None	National quarantine practices, first half of nineteenth century
International Governance	Horizontal strategies	Provides architecture for horizontal public health strategies	International Health Regulations
Global Governance	Vertical strategies	Provides norms that inform and guide vertical public health strategies	Global Fund to Fight AIDS, Malaria, and Tuberculosis

HORIZONTAL INTERNATIONAL REGIMES AND INFECTIOUS DISEASE CONTROL, 1851–1951

As Table B-1 indicates, before the mid-nineteenth century, states dealt with infectious disease problems solely through national governance. Each state adopted policies it thought best to deal with endogenous and exogenous disease threats without engaging in international cooperation. Processes of globalization—the increased volume and speed of international trade and travel—forced states to move from national to international governance in the mid-nineteenth century, and the 1851 International Sanitary Conference began the international governance endeavor on infectious diseases (Fidler, 2001b). As Table B-1 also indicates, international governance focuses primarily on horizontal strategies concerning the exportation and importation of infectious diseases. The first century of international health governance witnessed the creation of three primary horizontal international legal regimes relating to infectious diseases—the classical, organizational, and trade regimes.

The Classical Regime

The long line of international sanitary conventions adopted from the late nineteenth century until World War II (for a list of these treaties, see Fidler, 1999) and the International Sanitary Regulations (later renamed the International Health Regulations [IHRs] promulgated by the World Health

Organization (WHO) in 1951 constitute the *classical regime*. The IHRs' stated purpose—"to ensure the maximum protection against the international spread of disease with minimum interference with world traffic" (WHO, 1983)—captures the classical regime's objectives. The classical regime focuses solely on cross-border disease transmission by requiring (1) that states notify countries about cases or outbreaks of specified diseases in their territories and maintain adequate public health capabilities at points of disease exit and entry; and (2) that disease-prevention measures restricting or burdening international trade and travel be based on scientific evidence and public health principles.

The Organizational Regime

The second horizontal international legal regime is the *organizational regime*, which represents the various international health organizations (IHOs) created by states to deal with infectious diseases and other international public health problems. Today, WHO serves as the leading representative of the organizational regime. Although international law was central to the creation of IHOs, the treaties establishing them did not impose specific duties on states in terms of infectious disease control. States created IHOs to facilitate their horizontal cooperation on public health problems; but, in contrast with the classical regime, the organizational regime's legal duties for infectious disease control have been shallow at best.

The Trade Regime

The third major horizontal international legal regime, created during 1851–1951, was the *trade regime*, best represented by the General Agreement on Tariffs and Trade (GATT), adopted in 1947. The trade regime seeks to liberalize trade between states and thus is a classic example of horizontal interstate cooperation. The trade regime recognizes, however, that states may restrict trade to protect human health (GATT, Article XX[b]). Trade-restricting health measures to keep unsafe food from entering a country's market are, thus, legitimate if the state applying such measures follows the GATT disciplines on the issue. The trade regime represents, therefore, another horizontal international legal regime that contributes to international governance on infectious diseases.

GLOBALIZATION, INFECTIOUS DISEASES, AND CHANGES IN GOVERNANCE FRAMEWORKS AND STRATEGIES, 1951–2002

Globalization's impact on infectious disease control and prevention did not end in 1951 but has been ongoing. Many experts believe that globalization's influence on infectious diseases has accelerated in the past 10–15 years, as the literature on the crisis of emerging and reemerging infectious diseases suggests. The last 51 years have, however, witnessed changes in governance frameworks, the strategic emphasis of governance efforts, and the role of international law in the infectious disease context.

Shift in Focus from Classical to Trade Regime

The past half-century has seen the importance of the classical regime diminish and the importance of the trade regime grow. This shift from the classical to the trade regime can be seen in the intersection of two watershed events in horizontal international governance on infectious diseases. First, in 1995, WHO officially recognized that the IHRs had failed to achieve maximum protection from the international spread of disease with minimum interference with world traffic (World Health Assembly, 1995). WHO launched an effort to revise the IHRs to update their provisions for the new globalization challenges. Second, the World Trade Organization (WTO) came into existence in 1995 and quickly became the central horizontal regime for international law on infectious diseases. Two new trade agreements in the WTO—the Agreement on Trade-Related Aspects of Intellectual Property Rights (TRIPS) and the Agreement on the Application of Sanitary and Phytosanitary Measures (SPS Agreement)—combined to make the WTO more important in global public health circles than the IHRs, confirming that a shift from the classical to the trade regime had occurred.

IHR Revision: Rejuvenation or Death of the Classical Regime?

The shift described in the previous subsection raises many questions about the ongoing IHRs revision process. WHO's objective was to rejuvenate the IHRs to make the classical regime more robust and effective in the face of late twentieth century infectious disease threats. The IHR revision process may, however, be revealing the death of the classical regime.

The revised IHRs have the same objective as the existing IHRs: maximum protection against the international spread of disease with minimum interference with world traffic. To date, the revision process reveals a movement away from binding legal rules on disease notifications—one of the two fundamental legal pillars of the classical regime—to reliance on new global epidemiological information networks, represented by WHO's Global Outbreak Alert and Response Network (GOARN). WHO argues that GOARN has proven successful in helping WHO identify, verify, and investigate hundreds of infectious disease outbreaks since 1998. WHO notes that the outbreaks most frequently handled through GOARN have involved cholera, meningitis, haemorrhagic fevers, viral encephalitis, and anthrax. WHO claims that GOARN operates "within the framework of the International Health Regulations" (Heymann, 2002).

The WHO claim that the IHRs support GOARN is not correct from an international legal perspective. First, GOARN collects epidemiological data from governmental as well as nongovernmental sources. The IHRs authorize WHO to deal only with epidemiological information provided by the governments of member states (International Health Regulations, Part II, Articles 2–13). WHO's proposals to include in the revised IHRs the ability to collect data from nongovernmental sources demonstrate that the IHRs do not and cannot provide the legal foundation for GOARN's incorporation of nongovernmental information (see Fidler, 1999). Second, the IHRs address only three diseases—cholera, yellow fever, and plague (International Health Regulations, Article 1 [defining "diseases subject to the Regulations" as meaning cholera, plague, and yellow fever]). WHO recognized this limited coverage as being one of the major reasons why it needed to revise the IHRs (see Fidler, 1999). WHO's ability to deal, through GOARN, with meningitis, haemorrhagic fevers, viral encephalitis, anthrax, and other diseases not subject to the IHRs is not and cannot be supported by the IHRs.

WHO's claim that GOARN operates within the framework of the IHRs (Heymann, 2002) is also troubling because it contradicts the message WHO has been sending since 1995 that the IHRs are inadequate in the face of new globalization challenges. If the IHRs authorize WHO, through GOARN, to deal with nongovernmental sources of information and with a much longer list of infectious diseases, why did WHO argue from 1995 on that the IHRs are inadequate because they (1) do not allow use of nongovernmental epidemiological information, and (2) are severely constrained by applying to only three diseases?

The contradictory messages from WHO about the IHRs' relationship to GOARN is, to some extent, academic. What is more important is that GOARN operates on a large scale *without the revised IHRs being in place*. WHO notes that, between July 1998 and August 2001, it "verified 578 outbreaks of potential international importance in 132 countries, and investigated many hundreds more" (Heymann, 2002, p. 172). This fact suggests that WHO can pursue new approaches to global epidemiological surveillance based on new information technologies without the need for revised IHRs. This fact also suggests that revising the IHRs for purposes of global surveillance—the first raison d'etre of the classical regime—is not urgently required, or perhaps required at all.

The second objective of the IHRs is to achieve maximum protection against international disease spread *with minimum interference with world traffic*. WHO recognized in 1995—and much earlier for that matter (see, e.g., Delon, 1975; Dorelle, 1969; Roelsgaard, 1974)—that the IHRs had failed to prevent WHO member states from imposing irrational and unnecessary trade-restricting health measures. To date, nothing in the IHR revision process suggests that WHO member states want to strengthen WHO's hand against such irrational trade- and travel-restricting health measures. Today, the WTO provides the more important vehicle for states seeking to complain about irrational trade-restricting health measures because of the science-related and trade-related disciplines in the SPS Agreement. Thus, the second raison d'etre of the classical regime—discipline against irrational trade-restricting health measures—has migrated to the trade regime, at least for irrational health measures that restrict trade in goods.

Development of Vertical International Governance Regimes

In addition to the increased importance of the trade regime and the decreasing importance of the classical regime, the post–World War II period witnessed the development of new kinds of international governance regimes focused primarily on vertical strategies. Generally speaking, these three regimes seek to reform how a government interacts with its population health *inside the state's territory*. This section briefly describes the fundamental aspects of these three vertical international governance regimes.

Soft-Law Regime

The *soft-law regime* represents norms, guidelines, best practices, and policies generated by IHOs for adoption by states in their respective territories. The norms, guidelines, practices, and policies are not legally binding on the member states of the IHOs, which is why international lawyers describe this dynamic as involving "soft" rather than "hard" law. WHO has, for example, generated many such "soft-law" norms. In fact, WHO has preferred using soft-law norms to the creation of binding international legal commitments. The horizontal organizational regime has, thus, proven more valuable for vertical public health strategies than for disciplining interstate public health relations.

Environmental Regime

The *environmental regime* encompasses the body of international environmental law that states and international organizations have created largely in the post–World War II era (Birnie and Boyle, 2001). Much of international environmental law attempts to create rules that reduce environmental threats to human health, so this body of international law connects to public health (Fidler, 2001c). International environmental treaties often contain rules that require states to reduce environmental degradation within their territories and the cross-border transmission of environmentally harmful products and substances. International environmental law supports both horizontal and vertical strategies on environmental problems. International environmental law is, however, weakest in connection with vertical public health strategies against infectious diseases because this body of law does not address effectively local air and water pollution, which constitute the major environmental causes of infectious disease morbidity and mortality (Fidler, 2001c).

Human Rights Regime

International human rights law imposes obligations on governments in connection with their treatment of persons living in their territories (for the leading international human rights documents, see Brownlie, 1992). The focus of international human rights law, unlike that of international environmental law, is almost entirely vertical in orientation. Although international human rights law long incorporated public health issues, the emergence of the HIV/AIDS pandemic in the 1980s produced the first concerted effort to bring international human rights law to bear on public health policy and practices (Gostin and Lazzarini, 1997). Public health experts argued that international human rights law (1) protected persons living with HIV/AIDS from discrimination, and (2) imposed on governments obligations to respect, protect, and fulfill their citizens' human right to health by, for example, making prevention, testing, and treatment programs universally available. Compliance with international human rights law constituted a vertical public health strategy that sought to contribute to reducing infectious disease morbidity and mortality within a state.

Development of Global Governance Mechanisms and the Access Regime

The third major change seen in the post–World War II period is the development of global governance mechanisms. As described earlier, global governance involves the participation of states; intergovernmental organizations; and nonstate actors, such as MNCs and NGOs. The significant and often formal involvement of nonstate actors distinguishes global from international governance. Nonstate actors have long been involved in national and international governance, but experts perceive that globalization has produced new forms of global governance in which the nonstate actors take on more important governance functions. In the infectious disease context, we can discern various global governance mechanisms converging into what may be called the *access regime*—a vertical global governance regime that seeks to increase access to essential drugs and medicines for people living in developing countries.

Global Governance Mechanisms

Public health experts increasingly focus policy initiatives and academic research on "global health governance," with special emphasis on the growing roles of nonstate actors in the process of governance for public health (Dodgson et al., 2002, *supra* note 5). Perhaps the best example of this trend is the attention given to public–private partnerships, which have proliferated in the past decade in the context of global public health (Widdus, 2001). The role of nonstate actors in these global governance efforts ranges from formal to informal. The inclusion of NGO representatives on the governing body of the Global Fund to Fight AIDS, Malaria, and Tuberculosis (Global Fund) illustrates the formal incorporation of nonstate actors into a global governance mechanism (Global Fund, 2005). WHO's utilization of epidemiological information from nongovernmental sources in GOARN represents an informal incorporation of nonstate actors into a global governance mechanism. The new global governance mechanisms share common strategic ground in seeking to provide global public goods that states (especially developing countries) can utilize within their territories to reduce infectious disease morbidity and mortality. In other words, the new global governance mechanisms support primarily vertical public health strategies.

The Access Regime as Vertical Global Governance

Many global governance initiatives converge on a particular vertical strategy—increasing within developing countries access to drugs, vaccines, and other medicines for infectious diseases. Numerous public–private partnerships, such as the Global Alliance for Vaccines and Immunization (GAVI), the Global Alliance on Tuberculosis (GATB), and the Medicines for Malaria Venture (MMV), focus on developing and delivering new or existing drugs and vaccines more widely and effectively in developing countries. The Global Fund seeks to increase access to antiretroviral therapy in developing countries. The global movement to increase access to essential medicines can be seen as the evolution of a new regime—the access regime—that has become the most prominent and controversial development in the use of international law for infectious disease control purposes. This section briefly describes this emerging vertical global governance regime.

The access regime arose from the clash between the most prominent horizontal international governance regime—the trade regime—and the most prominent vertical international governance regime—the human rights regime. At the core of this clash was the collision of the TRIPS-led movement for greater protection for patented pharmaceutical products with human-right-to-health–inspired efforts to increase access to essential medicines in developing countries. The TRIPS versus public health battle produced the November 2001 adoption of the Declaration on the TRIPS Agreement and Public Health (WTO, 2001). The Declaration clearly supports placing public health objectives, especially access to medicines, above the trade-related goal of increasing patent protection for pharmaceuticals, and thus experts see it as a victory for the human-right-to-health movement and for public health governance generally.

One of the interesting themes of the development of the access regime is that major protagonists in the conflict were nonstate actors—pharmaceutical MNCs and NGOs (e.g., Médecins sans Frontières [MSF]). Nonstate actors also play significant roles in other aspects of the access regime, particularly through the various public–private partnerships that seek to develop new drugs for infectious diseases (e.g., MMV, GATB) or improve access to existing drugs (e.g., GAVI, Green Light Committee on Second-line TB Drugs). Nonstate actors also have a formal governance role in the Global Fund—another indication that the access regime represents an important development in global governance in the infectious disease context.

More conceptually, governance efforts to improve access to drugs and vaccines for infectious diseases are found within each framework of governance. Table B-2 describes some of these efforts.

TABLE B-2   The Access Regime and Governance Frameworks

National Governance	International Governance	Global Governance
NGO lawsuits filed in national court systems to force national governments to increase access to HIV/AIDS therapies under the precept of the human right to health (e.g., South African case of *Treatment Action Campaign v. Minister of Health* [December 2001])	Developing-country and WHO advocacy to strengthen the public health safeguards in TRIPS to ensure access to affordable drugs and medicines (e.g., Doha Declaration on the TRIPS Agreement and Public Health)	NGO activism directed at MNCs, international organizations, and national governments (e.g., MSF's global campaign opposing pharmaceutical MNCs' lawsuit against South Africa)
		Involvement of MNCs and NGOs in drug-development public–private partnerships
		Formal governance roles for nonstate actors in new institutions (e.g., Global Fund)

In essence, the access regime takes the human right to health, developed originally as a strategy of vertical international governance, into the realm of global governance through the leadership of nonstate actors. The access regime aims to develop not only governance frameworks at all levels conducive to improved access, but also new pharmaceutical products that governments, international organizations, and nonstate actors can deliver to people at the local level to reduce infectious disease morbidity and mortality.

The Access Regime and International Law

The development of the access regime indicates how international law's function in global governance differs from its role in international governance. Norms found in international law, principally the human right to health, inspire global governance activities on access, but international law does not provide the architecture for those activities. The various public–private partnerships, such as the Global Fund, are not based in treaty law, which is a classical international legal contribution to international governance. The participation of states and international organizations in these global governance efforts is, thus, nonbinding and voluntary as a matter of international law. From an international legal perspective, the access regime utilizes international law in ways very different from how states and international organizations have used international law for public health purposes since the beginning of international health diplomacy in 1851. Whether the access regime's use of international law signals a dramatic sea change in the relationship between international law and infectious disease prevention and control remains to be seen.

INFECTIOUS DISEASES AS FOREIGN POLICY AND NATIONAL SECURITY CONCERNS: GOOD FOR GOVERNANCE AND THE INTERNATIONAL RULE OF LAW?

The access regime represents one of the most prominent developments in infectious disease governance in the recent era of the globalization of public health. Another interesting development involves arguments that infectious diseases represent national security threats to the great powers and thus should be more important on their foreign policy agendas (see, e.g., Kassalow, 2001; Moodie and Taylor, 2000; NIC, 2000). In contrast to the movement toward vertical global governance seen in the access regime, these arguments seek to reconnect infectious disease control with national and international governance by reengaging the great powers in international public health. Should these arguments take hold, one might foresee reinvigorated national and international governance on infectious diseases to complement the developments in global governance.

Some caution is, however, advisable about arguments that infectious diseases represent national security and foreign policy threats. Historically, the great powers have not hesitated to bend, break, or abandon international law when they believed their national security was threatened. We can see this pattern in U.S. responses to the threat of biological weapons and bioterrorism. The United States has focused energy and new funding on homeland security against bioterrorism but has rejected multilateral efforts to strengthen international governance on the threat of biological weapons. Many see in these steps a rejuvenated U.S. unilateralism in an area in which public health plays a strategic role.

At the same time, the tepid and tardy responses of the great powers to the HIV/AIDS catastrophe in sub-Saharan Africa hardly serve as robust evidence that infectious disease problems in far-away countries have risen high on these nations' national security and foreign policy agendas. The shift from binding commitments in international governance to nonbinding, voluntary participation in global governance efforts may suit the narrow public health interests of the great powers to the long-term detriment of strengthening national and international governance on infectious diseases.

CONCLUSION

The globalization of public health creates infectious disease challenges that force states to engage in international cooperation. Historically, international law has been an important mechanism for facilitating international public health cooperation. International law's use in international infectious disease control connects to the governance challenges globalization presents in the public health context. This appendix has analyzed how states, international organizations, and nonstate actors have used international law for infectious disease control as part of the response to globalization challenges since the mid-nineteenth century.

The last 50 years, and the last decade particularly, have witnessed important shifts in how international law factors into infectious disease policy. Within the traditional realm of horizontal international regimes, attention has shifted from the classical to the trade regime. Attention has also shifted from horizontal international governance to vertical global governance. This latter shift finds the traditional function of international law in international governance overtaken by a context in which international law informs the creation of global governance endeavors that are not legally binding on any of the participants. As argued elsewhere (Fidler, 2001a, *supra* note 1), these new contexts mean that international law's role in infectious disease control today has never been more important and uncertain.

REFERENCES

Birnie PW, Boyle AE. 2001. *International Law and the Environment*. Oxford, UK: Clarendon Press.

Brownlie I, ed. 1992. *Basic Documents on Human Rights*. 3rd Ed. Oxford, UK: Oxford University Press.

Brownlie I. 1998. *Principles of Public International Law*. 5th Ed. Oxford, UK: Oxford University Press.

Delon PJ. 1975. *The International Health Regulations: A Practical Guide*. Geneva, Switzerland: WHO.

Dodgson R, Lee K, Drager N. 2002 (February). *Global Health Governance: A Conceptual Review*. Key Issues in Global Health Governance Discussion Paper No. 1. Geneva: WHO Department for Health in Sustainable Development.

Dorelle P. 1969. Old plagues in the jet age. *Chronicle of the World Health Organization* 23(3):103–111.

Fidler DP. 1999. *International Law and Infectious* Diseases. Oxford, United Kingdom: Clarendon Press. Pp. 22–23.

Fidler DP. 2001a. *International Law and Global Infectious Disease Control*, Commission on Macroeconomics and Health Working Paper No. WG2:18. [Online]. Available: http://www3.who.int/whosis/cmh/cmh_papers/e/pdf/wg2_paper17.pdf [accessed April 18, 2002].

Fidler DP. 2001b. The globalization of public health: The first 100 years of international health diplomacy. *Bulletin of the World Health Organization* 79(9):842–849.

Fidler DP. 2001c. Challenges to humanity's health: The contributions of international environmental law to national and global public health. *Environmental Law Reporter News and Analysis* 31(1):10048–10078.

Global Fund to Fight AIDS, Malaria, and Tuberculosis. *NGOs and Civil Society*. [Online]. Available: http://www.theglobalfund.org/en/partners/ngo/introduction/ [accessed September 12, 2005].

Gostin LO. 2001. *Public Health Law: Power, Duty, Restraint*. Berkeley, CA: University of California Press.

Gostin LO, Lazzarini Z. 1997. *Human Rights and Public Health in the AIDS Pandemic*. Oxford, United Kingdom: Oxford University Press.

Heymann DL. 2002. The microbial threat in fragile times: Balancing known and unknown risks. *Bulletin of the World Health Organization* 80(3):179.

Kassalow J. 2001. *Why Health is Important to U.S. Foreign Policy*. New York: Council on Foreign Relations and the CSIS International Security Program.

Moodie M, Taylor WJ. 2000.*Contagion and Conflict, Health as a Global Security Challenge*. Washington, DC: Chemical and Biological Arms Control Institute and the CSIS International Security Program.

NIC (National Intelligence Council). 2000. *The Global Infectious Disease Threat and Its Implications for the United States*. [Online]. Available: http://www.cia.gov/cia/publications/nie/report/nie99-17d.html [accessed March 27, 2002].

Roelsgaard E. 1974. Health regulations and international travel. *Chronicle of the World Health Organization* 28:265–268.

WHO (World Health Organization). 1983. *International Health Regulations*. 3rd Ed. Geneva, Switzerland: WHO.

Widdus R. 2001. Public-private partnerships for health: Their main targets, their diversity, and their future directions. *Bulletin of the World Health Organization* 79(8):713–720.

World Health Assembly. 1995 (May 12). *Revision and Updating of the International Health Regulations*. World Health Assembly Resolution 48.7. Geneva, Switzerland: WHO.

World Trade Organization (WTO). 2001 (Nov 14). *Declaration on the TRIPS Agreement and Public Health.* Ministerial Conference in Doha, Fourth Session, Nov 9-14, 2001. [Online]. Available: http://www.wto.org/english/thewto_e/minist_e/min01_ e/mindecl_ trips_e.htm [accessed September 13, 2005].

Appendix C

Changing Vector Ecologies: Political Geographic Perspectives

Jonathan D. Mayer, Ph.D.[1]

A ddressing only the changes in vector ecologies that have resulted from globalization is too narrow an approach for understanding the overall changes in disease ecology. If vector ecologies that are relevant to emerging infections are altered, the two relevant causal questions are how and why. Answers to these questions transcend biological factors. The crucial issue is to understand how changing social and human ecologies have interacted with alterations in vector ecologies to produce new patterns of disease. It is only through understanding social, environmental, and biological interactions that one can gain an understanding of static patterns or temporal changes in disease distribution. The Institute of Medicine's 1992 report on emerging infectious diseases (IOM, 1992) gave implicit credence to this argument, since five of the six factors in emergence (human demographics and behavior, technology and industry, economic development and land use, international travel and commerce, and breakdown in public health) are explicitly social in nature, and the sixth (microbial adaptation and change) is partly the result of social behavior and social change. However, social scientists have been minimally involved in research on emerging disease since 1992, and little social science has been incorporated into epidemiologic, public health, or infectious disease research and policy on emerging infections.

---

[1]Professor, Departments of Geography, Medicine (Allergy and Infectious Disease), Health Services, and Family Medicine, University of Washington, Seattle, Washington.

THE NATURE OF GLOBALIZATION

Globalization is a term often used in describing contemporary society, but it is frequently ill defined and misunderstood, and its definition is subject to argument. Indeed, its very conceptualization is "contested" (Buse and Walt, 2002, p. 42). It is frequently taken to mean the process of increasing global interdependency, but this is only part of the process of globalization as understood by contemporary social scientists. In the various descriptions and analyses of the effects of globalization that are found in the health sciences, interdependency, as manifested by increasing international transportation, is seen as the most salient feature that can affect the redistribution and movement of infectious disease. There is a fundamental tension that pervades both the popular and scholarly literature on globalization: globalization as a factor that promotes well-being and economic opportunity versus globalization as an alienating social force that marginalizes those at the periphery of societies.

What, then, is globalization? First, it is important to note that the health sciences could benefit from the explicit understanding of globalization as developed in international relations, political economy, political geography, and other disciplines. As noted in a recent article on the implications of the globalization of cholera for global governance: "an understanding of global health issues at the turn of the twenty-first century could benefit substantially from the voluminous literature on globalization from international relations, including the subfields of social and political theory and international political economy. This is a rich and voluminous literature. It documents what structural changes are occurring toward a global political economy, how power relationships are embedded within this process of change, what varying impacts this may have on individuals and groups..." (Lee and Dodson, 2000, p. 213). Clearly, then, globalization is something that is more profound than merely an increase in international interdependency and international connectivity. Moreover, changes in disease patterns that are the result of globalization are as old as globalization itself: many decades and perhaps centuries old, and the result of long-established historical transformations.

Globalization certainly contains elements of increasing global interdependency, the decline of international boundaries as deterministic social constructs, and the erosion of distance as an inhibitor of human interaction for some but not all segments of societies—though the effects of distance are highly variable, and some societies remain locally constrained. In addition, the term refers not only to increasing movement of goods and people or, as transportation geographers and regional scientists refer to such movement more generally, "spatial interaction," but also to the movement of capital. What is the movement of capital, and why is it relevant here? The movement of capital refers to the transferability of money, in its simplest sense, and to the increasing ties that characterize the world's financial system. The importance of this dimension of globalization is reflected in the fact that the "development of global financial markets" is Soros' (2002) operational definition of globalization. Thus, when an environmental project is financed in a country by funds from outside that country, it is the result of a global system of finance. This dimension has direct implications for local vector ecologies in the sense that a dam, for example, that is financed from outside the country, and perhaps even planned by a coalition of local and international environmental planners, may then alter the local breeding habitats of potential disease vectors, thereby changing the potential exposure to vectorborne or waterborne diseases.

Yet another dimension of globalization is changes in the locus of power in global decision making. One of the consequences of globalization, many argue, is that some localities are marginalized in their ability to control what happens to local society, and others are made more central and are able to project power over great distances. Society is seen as reflecting this reality in its increasing uniformity, erosion of locally controlled commodities and markets, and general loss of control. It is this dimension that is so politically controversial (e.g., Sassen, 1998) and is responsible for protests at the venues of organizations that are seen as representative of and as advocating increased globalization, such as the 1999 World Trade Organization meeting in Seattle. The process of globalization is nicely summed up by Joseph Stiglitz, former chief economist at The World Bank: "it is the closer integration of the countries and peoples of the world which has been brought about by the enormous reduction of costs of transportation and communication, and the breaking down of artificial barriers to the flows of goods, services, capital, knowledge, and (to a lesser extent) people across borders" (Stiglitz, 2002, p. 9).

THE SOCIAL ECOLOGY OF HUMAN DISEASE

Disease ecology explains infectious disease patterns in terms of the interactions of people and the environment. In the broadest sense, a social approach to disease ecology, even as conceived by May (1958), whose disease ecology was more medical than social, views infectious disease patterns as the result of cultural, social, behavioral, environmental, and biological interactions. In a dynamic sense, alterations in disease ecological relationships through environmental modifications therefore could be expected to alter human–vector relationships. The effects of land clearance projects, dam construction, and other environmental modifications can be seen in a number of examples.

Classic geographic disease ecology has developed incrementally since

World War II. Jacques May was a French surgeon in French Indochina who became intrigued by the interaction of local social and cultural patterns with equally local environmental conditions to produce patterns of contagion for a number of infectious diseases. He eventually gave up his surgical career to become the medical geographer at the American Geographical Society in New York City, where he produced numerous volumes and papers on disease ecology (e.g., May, 1958). As significant as his work was, he did not consider the impact of other regions on local conditions. Interregional patterns of commodity shipments, cultural contact, and cultural change are all aspects of global interdependency that were apparent decades ago. Moreover, May also did not consider the effects of power and politics on local disease conditions. Thus, disease ecology traditionally considered isolated regions in the absence of interaction, temporal change, and political power. The same framework saw fruition in the Soviet Union with the landscape epidemiology of Pavlovsky (1966) and his identification of local "nidi" of disease.

There are a number of examples of how globalization affects local disease ecologies and, by extension, human–vector interactions that are directly relevant to emerging infectious diseases. Most obviously, transportation is a benchmark of globalization because of the parallels between regional interdepedencies and the globalization phenomenon. Transportation moves commodities and people. Vectors may be unintentionally transported on either the transportation vehicle or the commodities that are being moved. An example of the former is the probable movement of anophelines from tropical to temperate areas and the occurrence of many instances of "airport malaria" surrounding major international airports, such as Detroit Metropolitan Airport, JFK Airport, Newark International, Amsterdam's Schiphol, London's Heathrow, and many others. An example of the transport of vectors on commodities is the introduction of the Asian tiger mosquito, *Aedes albopictus*, to the North American continent on rubber tires that were shipped to the port of Houston. *Ae. albopictus* is one of the vectors of dengue fever.

The movement of people is less subtle in the ways it can alter disease ecologies. Both short-term movement—travel—and longer-term movement—migration—are typical of globalization and have the potential to spread emerging infections. People may be infected with diseases endemic to one region and introduce those diseases to another region. This is almost certainly how HIV was introduced to North America, for example, and how fluoroquinolone-resistant gonococci were introduced from Asia.

A recent example of how movement may have introduced a new disease into a nonendemic area is the introduction of West Nile virus into North America. The most common vector of West Nile virus in the United States, the common household mosquito, *Culex pipiens*, was already ubiquitous in the New York metropolitan area. The mechanism of introduction is unclear, but it was probably through one of the following means: (1) movement of an infected individual into the New York City area; (2) movement of an infected bird, either via an airplane or other transportation vehicle or, less likely, via avian migration; (3) movement of an infected vector via airplane; or (4) shipment of an infected animal reservoir to the New York area. There may be no way to trace the precise means of introduction, but what is certain is that the disease was not present in North America until 1999 but was present on many other continents. Putatively, one may conclude that the infection came from elsewhere, almost certainly via transportation vehicle. The human–ecosystem relations were suitable in the New York metropolitan area to maintain the infection during the summer of 1999, and then to support its spread during subsequent summers via both human movement and bird migration.

THE POLITICAL ECOLOGY OF DISEASE

One of the useful ways of conceptualizing the impacts of decisions on local disease ecologies uses a combination of political economy and cultural ecology. Together they constitute the political ecology of disease (Mayer, 1996), and this construct has been applied to emerging infectious diseases (Mayer, 2000). These concepts require further explanation.

Political ecology more generally is "the attempt to understand the political sources, conditions, and ramifications of environmental change" (Bryant, 1992, p. 13). Thus, most broadly, the political ecological approach seeks to understand the unintended consequences of environmental decisions, and particularly those consequences that alter human–environment relations.

A dimension of globalization that is greatly emphasized in the social sciences but has received scant attention in the public health literature is the global flows of capital or, as Soros (2002) would have it, the internationalization of financial markets. There are many indirect consequences of this for public health, but the most direct consequence for emerging infections is that the flows of capital have financed projects that have altered human–environment relations at both the local and regional levels. Past examples of this are the construction of the Aswan Dam in Egypt and the Volta River Project in Africa. Unintended consequences of these large-scale water projects were the increased range and incidence of schistosomiasis, onchocerciasis, and malaria upstream of the dams. A more contemporary example is the construction and anticipated completion of the Three Gorges Dam in China. This massive project on the Yangtze River, designed explicitly for powering Chinese industrial growth and furthering China's position in the global economy, will almost certainly introduce schistosomiasis

(*Schistoma. japonicum*) into a nonendemic area upstream of the dam (e.g., Sleigh and Jackson, 1998; Xu et al., 1999). The ecological conditions will be conducive to schistosomiasis transmission, and there will be a great deal of human contact with the upstream lake—another case of the desire to be a more active participant in the world economy, and of the movement of global capital altering regional ecological conditions and affecting the transmission of emerging infections.

To generalize about the example of water projects that inevitably alter local vector ecologies, the purpose of these projects is usually to fuel economies through the generation of hydroelectric power. Typically, this has involved financing from outside the local area, providing an example of capital flows that affect disease transmission in more local areas. In the case of projects such as the Three Gorges Dam, financing is almost entirely from domestic sources (though some of that financing comes, indirectly, from business growth due to globalization), but a major purpose of the dam is to provide power to industries that will allow China to participate more fully in the global economy. Typically, there are unintended or unforeseen consequences for disease transmission or introduction in the local area that combine human patterns of interaction and behavior and biological parameters of vector habitat (Hunter et al., 1993). These general principles are not confined to water projects but are equally applicable to land clearance and other economic development projects that alter human–environment relations. For example, the land clearance in Malaysia that was done to permit the construction of rubber plantations, aimed at economic development and the promotion of an export economy, resulted in notable increases in malaria transmission among laborers on the plantation. This was due to the alteration in environmental conditions and vector ecology that made the landscape conducive to anopheline breeding and vastly increased contact by laborers with areas newly populated by anophelines (Meade, 1976).

GLOBAL WARMING AND VECTORBORNE DISEASE

In recent decades, many have noted the movement of vectors and alteration of vector ecologies not involving transportation. Of primary concern in this regard has been the movement of disease vectors, particularly malaria, as a result of global warming (Rogers and Randolph, 2000). Despite rhetoric to the contrary, however, any conclusions about whether global warming is actually causing increases in vectorborne disease prevalence or the movement of vectorborne disease into previously nonendemic areas are quite tentative.

The logic behind claims that global warming is increasing the range of vectorborne disease is quite appealing. Human activities, including industrialization, fossil fuel burning for heat and transportation, and deforestation cause global warming as a result of the increase of greenhouse gasses and the elimination of carbon sinks (through deforestation). The evidence for this is quite conclusive. It is equally certain that many aspects of vector behavior, including the range of habitability, are driven in part by temperature. Thus, it would appear reasonable to conclude that with global warming, the latitudinal range of tropical and subtropical vectors would move north in the northern hemisphere, south in the southern hemisphere, and higher in mountainous areas. In other words, many of the human activities that take place concomitantly with globalization appear to have the potential to alter the spatial distribution of vectors.

When subject to closer scrutiny, however, the situation is not as clear-cut. Multivariate mathematical and statistical models of transmission dynamics suggest that when variables in addition to temperature are included, the global incidence of malaria could actually decrease with global warming. This is due, in part, to the fact that rainfall would probably also increase, and local anopheline breeding areas would then be washed out. This would tend to override the effects of increased temperature. Moreover, some malarial vectors breed preferentially in warmer temperatures, and others prefer cooler temperatures and cannot even survive in warmer conditions; thus it is difficult to generalize about malaria, which is transmitted by dozens of anopheline species. Moreover, local ecological conditions are far more significant than the generalization of ecological conditions to a larger scale. Mathematical–spatial models are inevitably too coarse and lack sufficient geographic resolution. As Hackett observed in 1937: "Everything about malaria is so molded and altered by local conditions that it becomes a thousand different diseases and epidemiological puzzles. Like chess, it is played with a few pieces, but is capable of an infinite variety of situations" (Hackett, 1937, p. 266).

Adding to the uncertainty of whether global warming has increased vectorborne disease incidence is the fact that empirical studies have been contradictory. Some have correlated recent increases in malaria and dengue incidence with temperature increases, while others have found little or no change in incidence. One intriguing group of analyses used the El Niño Southern Oscillation (ENSO) to simulate, in the short term, longer-term climate changes. These studies then examined the effects of temperature and rainfall fluctuations on vectorborne disease incidence. Again, the results of these studies were contradictory. Moreover, because the weather fluctuations of ENSO are short-term, on the order of several years at the most, and global warming occurs over decades, the use of the ENSO phenomenon does not allow for the social adaptations to climate change that could mitigate its effects. As intriguing as the use of ENSO is as a surrogate for actual climate change, it does not mimic actual long-term changes in climate.

Thus, there is still uncertainty concerning the effects of climate change on vector ecologies and disease incidence. Existing mathematical models are not sophisticated enough to be truly predictive (NRC, 2001), and empirical studies are contradictory because the actual spatial patterns of disease that have occurred with climate change have been geographically variable, even under similar climatic conditions. This is probably because of the extreme sensitivity of local vector ecologies to local physical conditions and to human social and behavioral patterns. Few of the models and empirical studies have considered elements of social structure, demographic or settlement patterns, or human behavior. Rather, they have concentrated too narrowly on the physical and biological variables, and on simplistic deterministic models of vector behavior that are driven by temperature alone.

CONCLUSION

It is regrettable that there has been so little integration of social scientific concepts into the study of emerging infectious diseases, despite the fact the emergence of new diseases is due largely to social and geographic change. Rather, the vast preponderance of research and policy directed toward disease emergence has been explicitly biological in nature. What is necessary is a synthesis of biological, social, and political concepts to reach an overall understanding of emerging infections. This is particularly true in the context of globalization. One of the consequences of the lack of inclusion of social scientific understanding has been a restrictive definition of globalization in public health—an understanding that has included only the surface phenomena of transportation of people and commodities and of migration. Understanding the relationships between changing vector ecologies and globalization also necessitates an understanding of how political and economic decisions, particularly decisions that alter the landscape, in turn change human–environment relations in local and regional contexts.

REFERENCES

Bryant RL. 1992. Political ecology: An emerging research agenda in third world studies. *Political Geography* 11(1):12–36.
Buse K, Walt G. 2002. Globalisation and multilaterial public-private health parternerships: Issues for health policy. In: Lee K, Bruce K, Fustukian S, eds. *Health Policy in a Globalising World*. Cambridge, UK: Cambridge University Press. Pp. 41–62.
Hackett LW. 1937. *Malaria in Europe: An Ecological Study*. Oxford, UK: Oxford University Press.
Hunter JM, Rey L, Chu KY, Adekolu-John EO, Mott KE. 1993. *Parasitic Diseases in Water Resources Development: The Need for Intersectoral Negotation*. Geneva, Switzerland: WHO.
IOM (Institute of Medicine). 1992. *Emerging Infections: Microbial Threats to Health in the United States*. Washington, D.C.: National Academy Press.

Lee K, Dodson R. 2000. Globalization and cholera: Implications for global governance. *Global Governance* 6(2):213–236.

May JM. 1958. *The Ecology of Human Disease*. New York: M.D. Publications.

Mayer JD. 1996. The political ecology of disease as one new focus for medical geography. *Progress in Human Geography* 20:441–456.

Mayer JD. 2000. Geography, ecology, and emerging infectious diseases. *Social Science and Medicine* 50(7–8):937–952.

Meade MS. 1976. Land development and human health in West Malaysia. *Annals of the Association of American Geographers* 66:428–439.

NRC (National Research Council). 2001. *Under the Weather: Climate, Ecosystems, and Infectious Diseases*. Washington, D.C.: National Academy Press.

Pavlovsky EN. 1966. *The Natural Nidality of Infectious Disease*. Urbana, IL: University of Illinois Press.

Rogers and Randolph. 2000. The global spread of malaria in a future, warmer world. *Science* 289(5485):1763–1766.

Sassen S. 1998. *Globalization and Its Discontents*. New York: New Press.

Sleigh A, Jackson S. 1998. Public health and public choice: Dammed off at China's Three Gorges? *The Lancet* 351(9114):1449–1450.

Soros G. 2002. *George Soros on Globalization*. New York: Public Affairs.

Stiglitz J. 2002. *Globalization and Its Discontents*. New York: W.W. Norton.

Xu XJ, Yang XX, Dai YH, Yu GY, Chen LY, Su ZM. 1999. Impact of environmental change and schistosomiasis in the middle reaches of the Yangtze River following the Three Gorges construction project. *Southeast Asian Journal of Tropical Medicine and Public Health* 30(3):549–555.

Appendix D

Social Aspects of Public Health Challenges in Period of Globalization: The Case of Russia[1]

Andrey K. Demin, M.D., Doctor of Political Sciences, Candidate of Medical Sciences[2]

This research is based on variety of disciplinary perspectives, including political, social, and public health science, and attempts to add new approaches to and better understanding of global public health policy and governance at the national and international levels. The research methodology includes monitoring of public health and social security and relevant socioeconomic aspects, including activities implemented by the Russian Public Health Association, and comparative analysis of socioeconomic aspects of public health challenges. Some of the research materials were obtained by means of direct contacts with public health officials and experts and political scientists.[3] A search of available publications, including those on the Internet, was followed by structuring and analysis of the collected information and data.

[1]This research was carried out with support from the Bureau of Educational and Cultural Affairs of the U.S. Department of State and the Council for International Exchange of Scholars within the Fulbright New Century Scholars (NCS) Program for the academic year 2001–2002, "Challenges of Health in a Borderless World." Professor Ilona Kickbusch, director of the Division of Global Health in the Department of Epidemiology and Public Health at the Yale University School of Medicine, serves as the NCS distinguished scholar leader.

[2]President, Russian Public Health Association, and professor, Chair of Social Medicine, Economics and Administration of Health Care, I. M. Sechenov Moscow Medical Academy.

[3]A Fulbright scholar research visit to the Department of Global Health, School of Public Health and Health Services, the George Washington University Medical Center, Washington, D.C., in October–December 2002 was part of the NCS program. The author is grateful to Richard Southby, Ph.D., FCHSA, CHE, F.C.L.M. (Hon), Hon M.F.P.H.M., interim dean and Ross Professor of International Health; James E. Banta, M.D., M.P.H., FACPM, interim chair; and the staff of the department for their support.

This paper addresses in turn Russia in a globalizing world; public health theory and practice in Russia; public health challenges in Russia; political, economic, and social factors related to public health challenges in Russia; and the role of various political actors in public health. The final section presents conclusions.

RUSSIA IN A GLOBALIZING WORLD

Since the 1990s, globalization has become dominant in the world arena.[4] Globalization is an objective reality in international relations, with an attendant political model, leaders, logic, and institutional system (Dakhin, 2001). The place of Russia in the changing political and economic world order is an important issue. Dissolution of the USSR and the Soviet bloc proved that the previous political, social, and economic systems were exhausted. Responses to the challenges of the postindustrial era were inadequate because of political and information secrecy, state control of information, and the absence of markets. These obstacles were removed in post-Soviet Russia after 1991. Since then, the country has been in search of a new paradigm of progress and development that involves joining the globalized economy, as well as internal stability and development.

Efforts aimed at preservation of the post–World War II world order, proclaiming post-Soviet Russia as successor to the former superpower, proved to be futile. According to the National Security Concept of the Russian Federation, adopted in January 2000 (Concept of National Security of Russian Federation, 2000), in the postbipolar period, the national interest in the international sphere is in ensuring sovereignty and strengthening Russia's position as a great power—one of the influential centers of the multipolar world. However, there is also a countertrend toward construction of a unipolar world dominated by developed western countries, with U.S. leadership in the international community, and envisaging unilat-

---

[4]Globalization is described as a stage in internationalization of social relations beyond the borders of nation-states at the global level, increasing interdependence of states and regions (Matveevskiy); the process of developing a single global financial and information space on the basis of computer technologies (Delyagin, 2001); increasing transparency of nation-state borders for flows of capital, information, and population migration. Geopolitical and geoeconomic zones, previously closed for capital and information flows, are opened. Globalization became possible with the victory of capital and freedom of information over national interests. Capital is losing its national identity. On the global scale, financial capital gains a victory over industrial capital (Kargalitsky, 2001). Transnational corporations are believed to be the driving force of globalization. They are supported by the governments of the countries leading globalization, and indirectly by international trade and financial organizations dominated by these countries (Matveevskiy) Economic activity becomes increasingly independent from the state, which loses the ability to manage its own economic and social affairs.

eral, military-first solutions of the key issues of world politics and circumventing the basic norms of international law.

Russian scholars (Dakhin, 2001) argue that the latter trend prevails, and that economic globalization has become an instrument in the construction of such a unipolar model of world order, in which sovereignty is limited. This political model has thus far failed to encompass the whole world. Domination of financial markets and recurrent financial crises may compromise the neoliberal approach promoted by national governments and international financial institutions such as the World Trade Organization (WTO), the International Monetary Fund, and The World Bank, and the world economy may turn to greater use of state regulation (Kargalitsky, 2001).

Russian experts (Fedotova, 2001) claim that after the dissolution of the USSR, countries leading the globalization process became indifferent to the social quality of non-Western societies unless it threatened relevant interests. The goals of integration into the global economy were separated from the goals of internal development.

The negative impact of the current pattern of globalization is becoming more pronounced in a number of countries, including developed ones (Bezruchka, 2000), as a result of environmental decline; marginalization of specific regions and social groups, such as youth, the aged, and employees of declining branches of the economy; and liberalization of social policy. In response to the unipolar political model, antiglobalist sentiment takes the form of social clashes, extremism, and terrorism (Dakhin, 2001). Inequalities in development are generating tension in international relations.

One of the features of transnational social organization is the freedom of movement of individuals beyond national borders. Thus issues of health and social security become international and necessitate the development of transnational and global health policy and governance (Kickbusch and Buse, 2001; Kickbusch and de Leeuw, 1999; Lee, 1999). Public health challenges become a basic element in the stability of international political systems. This is important from the point of view of the prevention and control of infectious disease (IOM, 1997).

Many of the critical issues related to global health[5] and increasing global interdependence are represented in post-Soviet Russia, and globalization can provide keys to some solutions. It is a positive movement to-

---

[5]Demographic destabilization; accelerating developmental disparities; health-in-development strains; health-in-prosperity strains; persistent underattention to the vulnerabilities and capabilities of girls and women; infrastructural inadequacy and inappropriateness; deficiencies of cooperation, coordination, and governance; facilitation of biomedical research; facilitation of clinical practice; microenvironmental problems; environmental degradation; demand for personally and socially harmful substances; violence (Koop et al., 2000).

ward economic and social progress (Matveevskiy) including public health advancement. Globalization can help overcome the negative aspects of development. It is impossible for any state to develop in isolation. However, a political model of globalization should serve the broader interests of the global community, primarily those related to environmental, social security, and public health challenges. Global policy and governance in the interests of all states and nations, based on relevant institutional and legal components, is needed in the era of global interdependence, when "Everyone is responsible to everyone for everything."[6]

It should be noted that post-Soviet Russia emerged at the peak of a political, socioeconomic, and public heath crisis, and since then has been an object rather than a subject of globalization (Dakhin, 2001). The choice of a neomodernization model by the ruling elite in the era of globalization, along with economic weakness and other factors, brought the country to the periphery of the globalizing world (Fedotova, 2001).

In the 1990s, a radical approach to change aimed at transfer of the Western institutional model was combined with demodernization as a result of the inappropriateness of the selected model of development to the culture of the population. In brief, Russia "returned" to obsolete or nonexistent values as a result of the dominance of demodernization with elements of Westernization. As a result, in the 1990s there developed in Russia a form of "crony" or "wild" capitalism different from the Western model, lacking a labor basis and the ethics of entrepreneurship. Neomodernism was discredited. The challenge of internal social development was further complicated in Russia by recurrent debate on the Eurasian concept.

An important factor is that until recently, the majority of Russian politicians and scholars overlooked and misinterpreted globalization. Attitudes toward globalization have been dominated by black-and-white sentiments, an approach traditional for the Russian social sciences. Globalization has often been understood ideally, as a global conspiracy against the USSR and Russia, the forced opening of the country, the loss of its global role, the destruction of national "goods," and the importation of global "bads." With a few exceptions (Russian Federation, 2000), discussion of globalization and Russia has centered on WTO accession and its impact on the economic interests of specific narrow groups.

The unprecedented economic openness of post-Soviet Russia does not imply its integration into the globalized economy, for several reasons. The first is economic weakness and the decline of research. The USSR and its

---

[6]This formula of global interdependence and social justice was developed by Russian writer and philosopher Fedor Dostoyevsky in the nineteenth century.

allies made up a powerful single unit of economic space and a part of the world economy. That space was split after the dissolution of the USSR. Post-Soviet Russia does not possess an economic complex; rather, it is a geoeconomic vacuum without an autonomous identity in the world (Dakhin, 2001). Currently the country's share of global trade is small, and it is dominated by raw materials. Russia's prospects are compromised by a huge international debt, considerable uncontrolled outflow of capital, and weak regional integration.

Views on Russia entering the globalized economy vary from optimistic to pessimistic. Yet this is an urgent challenge, and breakthrough strategies as well as adequate internal development are needed. Nationalist sentiments and further social disintegration or a social explosion after a period of apathy are possible in the current circumstances. However, a postmodernist option is still possible for Russia.

Russia might be considered an ideal place for the development of ideologies that could serve as an alternative to globalism because the latter does not possess a social basis, the old ideology has been destroyed, and a new one has not emerged. However, continuing systemic crises promote antiglobalist protest (Dakhin, 2001).

A number of projects for the future development of Russia have been put forward by representatives of the elite. However, isolation of the elite has always been typical for Russia. The Russian elite is challenged to determine the character of the Russian state as a new entity with new political and economic systems, values, and ideology, or as an "echo" of the USSR. On that basis, the system of national interests and their hierarchy according to political and economic realities should be developed, ideologically based, and protected if Russia is to secure a sound place in the changing world, including participation in the development of new approaches for a global world order, public health policy, and governance.

PUBLIC HEALTH THEORY AND PRACTICE IN RUSSIA

Analysis of the development of public health theory and practice in Russia, closely related to the political, economic, and social changes in the country, is also important for understanding the country's public health challenges and response.

From the 1917 Socialist Revolution until the late 1920s, the theoretical approach taken was termed "social hygiene." It was highly political and directly connected to revolutionary practice and the construction of a new society and state, and it combined Marxism, hygiene, sociology, and prerevolution achievements in population health (Field, 1992; Kazan, 1998).

Soviet social hygiene provided a basis for the development of a new system of health protection and improvement. It was also used as a means for increasing the loyalty of health professionals, incorporating education in Marxist philosophy and related social sciences. Enrollment of new medical students increased considerably. However, a "class approach" was practiced in the training of medical professionals.[7] Soviet social hygiene claimed that diseases and premature mortality are the product of a "sick" capitalist social system, social habits, and institutions, and that population health would be improved with the advent of "healthy" socialism and ultimately communism through the transformation of society and the education of the population.

From the late 1920s, Soviet social hygiene was suppressed by the ruling political elite. Communist Party decisions to implement industrialization under a forced draft and collectivization of agriculture on the basis of administrative-and-command management further exacerbated social conditions, and the former official approach to population health became inappropriate. Public health theory and the health care system were shifted toward the classic clinical approach. Information on many population health indices was suppressed, as was international collaboration in public health. In 1929 the "class approach" was proclaimed as a principle of health care.

From 1941 until the mid-1960s, public health science was further reduced and officially termed the "organization of health care." It had to execute command and administrative decisions and to prepare dogmatic, unsubstantiated recommendations (Kazan, 1998).[8] Foreign public health research and practice were largely ignored or criticized as irrelevant to the Soviet system.

A postwar campaign to control cosmopolitism, eradicate bourgeois influence, and prove the universal priority of domestic and Soviet science included debates among specialists on social hygiene versus organization of health care. Social hygiene was viewed by many as "the Western, reformist, cosmopolitan and bourgeois science." Many distinguished specialists were repressed.

In the early 1950s, a dogmatic attitude toward health care as the "nonproductive" sphere in the national economy emerged. In 1966, the official term for public health science was changed to "social hygiene and organization of health care."

---

[7]New medical students were selected according to their "class origin," almost exclusively among the children of workers and peasants, based on the ideological postulate of the primacy of the proletariat and the peasantry as its ally (Kazan, 1998).

[8]For example, it was postulated that socialism is free from conflict among social classes; thus population health does not depend on social conditions and factors. This view mixed class and social categories and compromised public health science in the USSR (Kazan, 1998).

Soviet public health theory and practice were increasingly unable to address the unfolding epidemic of noncommunicable diseases and relevant risk factors, as well as "social" diseases, including abuse of psychoactive substances (tobacco, alcohol, and drugs) and sexually transmitted diseases (STDs) (e.g., HIV/AIDS). Informed discussion of public health challenges as a basis for developing policy response was impossible for specialists, the media, or concerned citizens. Neglect of public health theory and research, as well as of the social costs of political and economic decision making, continued.

Extensive development of the health care system was undertaken. The numbers of hospital beds and physicians were increased, despite shortages of resources, without due consideration for quality of care. The health system was characterized by neglect of economic incentives in health care, medicalization of care, and use of administrative and command approaches to handling public health issues and did not meet promises of universal free care. Salaries of medical professionals as state employees were kept low, and they were deprived of the right to establish independent associations. Women came to represent the majority (70 percent) of the profession (except the administrative elite).

Among the historical successes of Soviet public health theory and practice is the invention of the state model of the health care system in 1919; its principles and practices were later used in many countries. The Soviet system proved to be effective in the prevention and control of infectious disease. During the Great Patriotic War (1941–1945), the health system returned to military duty more than 72 percent of the wounded and 90 percent of ill soldiers and officers. By 1940, provision of beds and physicians was close to that in the economically developed world, and it has further improved since then. By the mid-1960s, Russia's public health profile was comparable to that of many Western countries. The comprehensive health and social security of the Soviet citizen was considered by many to be an international "yardstick."

However, public health theory and practice failed to prevent the decline of many public health indicators, experienced in Soviet Russia after 1964, with a short period of relative improvement in 1985–1987 with the advent of "perestroika." This decline can be explained largely by the sacrificing of social to military concerns during the cold war (Field and Twigg, 2000).[9]

---

[9]In the post–World War II period, the USSR, possessing economic potential considerably below that of the United States, started to accumulate and attempted to maintain a comparable military destructive potential in a bipolar world-order setting. The social cost of the effort was enormous, and a comprehensive public health decline began. The western Siberian oil and gas fields have provided up to 50 billion U.S. dollars annually since the 1970s. These mammoth resources were spent for the implementation of military programs, including nuclear and space programs, compensation of ineffective agriculture, and other "projects of the cen-

It should be noted that loss of life and health in the country was profound after 1917. The impact of World War I (1914–1918); the radical changes in the Russian political, social, and economic systems; dissolution of the Russian Empire; and the transition to socialism resulted in a demographic disaster.[10] The human toll of industrialization and collectivization was great.[11] Repressive political regimes increased the losses.[12] About 27 million died during the Great Patriotic War (1941–1945).

During the post-Soviet period, substantial changes took place in public health theory and practice. Health information was declassified in 1993; modern research became possible, international collaboration began to develop, and activities of international players in Russia commenced.

Attempts to modernize public health theory and practice according to Western approaches began. Since the introduction of health insurance in 1991, however, the economic model for medical care provision and administrative issues has been the focus of attention of reformers. As a result of a decline in funding of science and education, a "gold fence" succeeded an "iron fence" in the development of public health theory and practice.

Public health science became politicized. Positive and negative impacts of globalization on public health were not considered adequately. The approach to public health in social policy reduced health to survival; the importance of the absence of disease and subjective individual satisfaction with or control over factors influencing health were overlooked. A "multi-layer" health care system developed, compromising social justice. The decline was further exacerbated after 1991, with a short period of improvement in 1995–1998.

In 2000, the challenge of depopulation and inadequate social security, including health care, was positioned as a priority at the highest political level by the President of the Russian Federation, Vladimir Putin. The official term for public health science was changed to "public health and health care," and attempts to modernize the approach continued. Thus Russia is

---

tury," but not for improving the health of the population. In the 1970s the state further suppressed information on some deteriorating health and demographic indices.

[10]Civil war, war with Poland, war in Central Asia, foreign military intervention, disease, and a major famine in 1917–1922 caused about 12.5 million excess deaths in Russia in 1918–1922. An estimated 2–3.5 million people emigrated from the country (Ellmann, 2000).

[11]Famine in the former USSR in 1933 claimed more than 7 million lives, including more than 2 million in Russia.

[12]It is estimated that until the 1950s, there were more than 20 million inmates in the former USSR GULAG system. In 1941–1945 in the camps and prisons, about 1 million men and over 100,000 women perished. Approximately 3 million "repressed peoples" were subjected to forced deportation. About 800,000 "special settlers" died during transportation and the first years of life in the new, severe circumstances. These situations were typical for Russia.

able to participate in the development of global public health policy and governance by the global public health community on a common theoretical and practical basis.

PUBLIC HEALTH CHALLENGES IN RUSSIA

The public health decline after 1991 exacerbated the long-term trend that emerged in 1964. Among major public health challenges in Russia are depopulation, high mortality, low birth rates, intensive migration (including illegal), increasing morbidity, and the rise of infectious diseases such as tuberculosis (TB) and AIDS. The global importance of these public health challenges should be emphasized. They can change the geopolitical landscape dramatically in a relatively short period of time (CIA, 2001). Indeed, some alarmist forecasts question the existence of the Russian nation in the next century.

The increase in mortality from 1988–1994 was the beginning of a long-term negative trend. As noted, a short period of improvement was confined to 1995–1998. The global trend among the majority of developed countries toward falling fertility and aging is combined in Russia with high mortality, resulting in population decline.

The death rate is 1.7 times the birth rate. The excess of deaths over births in 1992–2000 reached 6.8 million, and the total population in 2001 had decreased to 145 million. Depopulation has become a national challenge. However, the phenomenon should be confirmed by the population census of October 2002 because of inadequate data on immigration during the period after the 1989 census (immigration may have compensated for the excess of deaths over births).

The birth rate decreased by a factor of 1.6 in 1990–2000, down to 8.7 per 1,000. The death rate had increased to 15.3 per 1,000 by 2000. The average life expectancy in 2000 was only 59.0 years among men and 72.2 among women (Government of the Russian Federation, 2001a). There has been a considerable decline in fertility. In 1988–1998, the net reproduction rate and the total fertility rate fell by 42 percent, leading to a sharp population decline (Ellmann, 2000). About 20 percent of couples suffer from infertility.

Fitness for military service among conscripts has declined (Gerasimenko, 1997). Abuse of psychoactive substances (tobacco, alcohol, and narcotics) has increased. In 1987–1999, the proportion of smokers among men in the age group 30–39 increased from 51 to 71 percent. The number of 15- to 17-year-old teenagers registered at narcotics dispensaries as drug users increased 12 times.

Demographic challenges are more qualitive than quantitive in nature. There are many indicators of decline:

• Declines in somatic and mental health are accompanied by increases in TB, syphilis, and AIDS.

• According to expert assessment, 70 percent of the population experiences long-term psychoemotional and social stress, resulting in increases in depression, reactive psychoses, and neurotic disorders.

• Social ill health is characterized by high levels of alcohol abuse, drug abuse, and suicide.

Especially distressing is the decline in maternal and child health. Health problems have increasingly shifted from the elderly to children and youth. Each succeeding generation possesses worse health and lower life expectancy. Ill generations fail to produce healthy offspring, and this may imply a long-term decline in the human potential of the nation. In spite of their higher life expectancy relative to men, women's individual health potential is lower than men's. Poor health of women results in the birth of unhealthy children. In 1996, over one-third of pregnant women suffered from anemia, and one-third of children were born unhealthy. Only 10 percent of children finishing school are healthy, and only one-third of conscripts are fit for military service.

The role of infectious disease in declining living standards and other social factors, especially poverty, is rising. TB, responsible for over 80 percent of deaths from infectious and parasitic diseases, caused 29,600 thousand deaths in 2000. The incidence of TB stabilized at 87.3 per 100,000 in 2001. Among inmates, its incidence is 35 times higher, and mortality from the disease is much higher as well. STDs have also increased. For example, in 1990–1997 the incidence of syphilis increased 64 times, up to 277.7 per 100,000, although it had decreased by 40 percent by 2000. Hospital infections are also on the rise. The incidence of HIV is high as well; more than 55,000 new cases were registered in 2000. Viral hepatitis, especially hepatitis B, is also increasing (Government of the Russian Federation, 2001a). In the early 1990s, there was an epidemic of diphtheria due to a decline in immunizations in 1990–1991; it was brought under control by 1995.

Migration has become a very important issue for Russia. The total number of migrants in Russia according to the United Nations is 13 million. Only in the United States is the number of foreign migrants higher with 35 million migrants (United Nations, 2002). There is a considerable inflow of migrants from the states of the former USSR. This migration is not monitored or controlled from an epidemiological point of view because of a lack of funds and is thereby posing a threat.

According to some forecasts, by 2010 the number of illegal migrants into Russia could increase to 19 million, representing 15 percent of the total population. The current number of illegal migrants according to various estimates is 5.5–12 million (Korich, 2002). Illegal migration from China, Afghanistan, Iran, Iraq, and other countries takes place. Many migrants come from countries with unfavorable sanitary–epidemiological profiles. Temporary work accounted for 300,000 migrants in 2001. The majority of these migrants are employed in production and transportation, and many do not pay taxes.

Since 1990, 1000,000 individuals have emigrated from the country for permanent residence abroad each year (Government of the Russian Federation, 2001a). Finally, in 2001 Russia was visited by 21.5 million foreigners, including 7.4 million tourists.

POLITICAL, ECONOMIC, AND SOCIAL FACTORS RELATED TO PUBLIC HEALTH CHALLENGES IN RUSSIA

In Soviet Russia, state social programs were the sole provider of safety nets for the population. These programs, as well as the economy and industry, were fueled until 1992 largely by state exports of natural resources, not manufacturing. Thus in principle, the labor force was of secondary importance for the satisfactory functioning of the Soviet model. Nevertheless, the social security of Soviet citizens (setting aside its quantity and quality) was more comprehensive compared with developed welfare states according to the "Soviet social contract."

The dissolution of the USSR and the shift away from a bipolar world compromised "Soviet civilization" as a global phenomenon, with profound repercussions for public health. A change in the model of political and socioeconomic development necessitated new approaches to addressing public health issues. However, the ruling elite failed to meet this challenge. In accordance with the neoliberal approach, the state deserted the social policy arena. "Shock therapy" wiped out savings. Privatization and the market failed to substitute for Soviet state safety nets destroyed by the "two nations" reform project. The bulk of the population was deprived of economic power and thus became "excessive" at this stage of post-Soviet reform. Russia is a highly urbanized and relatively cold country (40 percent of the total area consists of permafrost regions); thus a considerable portion of households could not switch to private gardening as the basis for their subsistence.

Rhetoric aside, the practical indifference of the post-Soviet Russian elite and the state toward social policy and public health issues in 1991–1999 might be explained by the emphasis on the redistribution of state property inherited from the USSR, the control over flows of funds generated in the sphere of natural resource use, the allocation of budgetary funds and foreign loans, and adaptation to changes in the place of Russia in the world. As noted, the importance of population for the elite and for the acceptable functioning of the state bureaucracy further diminished during that period: final product represented less than nine percent of Russia's total exports. Another argument supporting this point is the lack of effective action of the state until 2000 on collecting taxes, as well as later introduction of a 13 percent flat-rate income tax. The population demonstrated high tolerance to hardships and the level of protest was low, despite the fact that the structure of the country's gross national product might imply the right of every individual to receive considerable benefits based on the fact of citizenship alone. A decline in production, abolition of the state monopoly on foreign trade, natural resources, and alcohol turnover, and biased privatization of state property created a small, deindustrialized, raw material export–oriented economy beneficial for a small segment of the population and promoting outflow of capital.

Currently, Russia is in rather a geoeconomic vacuum. Its gross domestic product (GDP) is less than two percent of the world GDP. External debt stands at $US 138.1 billion. A considerable portion of the state budget is allocated to servicing this debt. Internal debt is high. Foreign investment in Russia in 1992–1998 totaled $US 15.9 billion (Russian Federation, 2000), comparable to an outflow of capital in one year (2001) of $US 17 billion.

Positive changes took place in post-Soviet Russia, related to ensuring political freedoms, opening up the society, effecting political and administrative reform, and developing market relations. The availability and variety of consumer goods and services increased as a result of price and trade liberalization. Cultural, economic, and recreational benefits were derived from increased foreign travel. The variety of media increased, and the Internet became accessible. Opportunities for legal self-employment and entrepreneurship increased and were seized by millions of people (Ellmann, 2000; Rimashevskaya, 1998a).

Public health challenges develop in parallel with, though lag behind, changes in the economy and social security. This was illustrated by a decline in public health in 1992–1994 and after the August 17, 1998, economic crisis in Russia; the latter resulted in a four-fold devaluation of the national currency. A considerable portion of the Russian population became involved in the vicious circle of poverty, disease, and premature death.

One of the first results of the post-Soviet changes was rapid impoverishment: from 1987–1988 to 1993–1995, the total number of poor increased from 2.2 to 57.8 million; 10 percent of the impoverished are considered the social "bottom" and are rejected by the society (Rimashevskaya, 1998b). According to official statistics, the share of population with incomes less than the living minimum is approximately 30 percent (Ellmann, 2000). In 1992–1996, the highest incidence of poverty was among children under six.[13] There are at least one million neglected and homeless children. Impoverishment has resulted in

---

[13]By 1997, up to half of children under 18 were among the urban poor. Stunting in children under age two increased from 9.4 percent in 1992 to 15.2 percent in 1994.

large-scale undernourishment (Rimashevskaya, 1998b) and increasing morbidity and mortality.

In 1990–1999, formal-sector employment fell sharply (UNECE, 2000a). The result was a decline in individual and family income, social exclusion, and declining life opportunities for children. Official employment was characterized by a large-scale failure to pay wages regularly in money and in full.[14] Registered unemployment increased in 1994–1999 from 7.5 to 12.3 percent (Goskomstat estimates according to the International Labor Organization definition) (UNECE, 2000b).

Morbidity and mortality from diseases associated with poverty and unemployment increased. The greatest decline in fertility was seen in regions of the "rust belt," which also experienced the greatest fall in industrial production and the highest unemployment, suggesting that the worsening economic circumstances since 1989 forced people not to have children. This point is further confirmed by a decline in the mean age of childbearing (Ellmann, 2000).

The increase in mortality was highest among men of working age, and was sometimes related to alcohol abuse (Shkolnikov and Nemtsov, 1997). Increased alcohol consumption is explained by a decline in its relative price and unrestricted accessibility. State and social control of alcohol use deteriorated in 1987 after the anti-alcohol campaign ended. The state alcohol monopoly was abolished in post-Soviet Russia at the end of 1991 by neoliberal ministers, sacrificing public health and state tax income to market interests. State officials also created opportunities for the penetration of the transnational tobacco, alcohol, and beer industries into the country. It should be noted that abuse of alcohol and other psychoactive substances is a traditional "escape from reality" when a response to intensive stress is needed (Bezruchka, 2000).

Inequality in wealth is leading to an increasing inequality in health. By 1995 the average income of the richest 20 percent was 8.5 times higher than that of the poorest 20 percent of the population (Rimashevskaya, 1998a).[15]

The winners in the process of change are those who are young, in good health, well educated, flexible, entrepreneurial, and mobile, and those who have privileged access to enterprise assets. The social groups that have borne the social costs of the change process are industrial workers and budget-sector employees, children, women, refugees, and persons displaced because of social and military conflicts. Men constitute the majority among both the beneficiaries and victims of change. Lifestyle factors have promoted gender gaps in mortality and life expectancy (Ellmann, 2000).

---

[14]Due to wage arrears, payment in kind, administrative leave, involuntary part-time and short-time work, extended maternity leave, and early retirement.

[15]It is known that social stability is threatened if the difference is more than 10–12-fold (Rimashevskaya, 1998b).

After the breakup of the USSR, about 25 million Russians remained in the New Independent States outside Russia. Their status was reduced to that of ethnic minority, and in many states they were deprived of basic rights and discriminated against. Some emigrated to Russia.

A very inexpensive or free network of public services (e.g., medical care, education, sport, public housing, public transport, garbage collection, preschool child care, cinemas, theaters) ceased to exist because of budget cuts or privatization. This development negatively affected a large proportion of the poor, especially pensioners, the disabled, and orphans.[16]

Scholars emphasize the important role of stress related to the failure of the state in Russia's increased mortality. This stress results from the destruction of behavioral stereotypes and adaptation to changed roles and circumstances, reduced incomes, the loss of safety nets, and so on (Field and Twigg, 2000; Shapiro, 1995).

Post-Soviet changes led to increases in socioeconomic pathologies: corruption; criminalization; and alcohol, tobacco, and drug abuse. The criminalization of society has prevented social and economic development. Close links among the criminal, political, and business worlds have developed. Growth in corruption, including bribes and theft of public money, resulted from state failure, the rotation of elites, and the inadequate introduction and enforcement of legal and cultural norms and values. This in turn affected efficiency, policies, distribution, incentives, and the political system (Ellmann, 2000).

In 2001 there were two million inmates in Russia, and three million criminal offences were registered.[17,18] Each year 30,000 individuals are reported lost. Russia ranks second in the world in homicide incidence, after South Africa. According to Transparency International, in 2001 Russia was 79th among 91 groups of countries on the corruption perception index, the degree to which corruption is perceived to exist among public officials and politicians.[19] Moreover, post-Soviet armed conflicts resulted in loss of life, injuries, migration, and damage to property.

It is obvious that the hasty opening of the country to globalization processes during a crisis in social development has been one of the key factors in public health changes. Examples of these agents of change are

---

[16]Basic educational enrollment (as the percentage of the 7–15 age group) declined during 1989–1998 from 93 to 87.5 percent. Educational opportunities are diminishing for rural populations, the less affluent, and the less well connected, who are at risk of social exclusion (Ellmann, 2000). The Russian health care system was ranked 130th among 191 countries (WHO, 2000).

[17]For further information go to www.vokruginfo.ru/news/news1921.html.

[18]There are two million officers within the Ministry of Internal Affairs system.

[19]For further information go to www.transparency.org/cpi/2001/cpi2001.html.

shifts in social values; outflow of capital; intensified migration; internation-alization of crime; devaluation of the national currency in 1998; and large-scale imports of falsified food, alcoholic beverages, pharmaceuticals, toys, and other goods. Transnational producers of global "bads" such as to-bacco, alcohol, and "junk food" penetrated Russia after 1991, using the window of opportunity provided by globalization processes. Currently, transnational companies control about 65 percent of local tobacco produc-tion. Tobacco production increased in 1990–2001 from 150.5 to 398 bil-lion cigarettes (Gerasimenko and Demin, 2002). Beer consumption has been increasing by 25–30 percent annually. The world center of illegal drugs has moved closer to Russia, to Afghanistan.

ROLE OF VARIOUS POLITICAL ACTORS IN PUBLIC HEALTH

Four actors shape public health policy in the era of globalization: the state, private enterprises, civil society, and international players.

Development of state public health policy in post-Soviet Russia can be divided into two periods. The first is Boris Yeltzin's presidency in 1992–1999. A law introducing compulsory and obligatory medical insurance was adopted in 1991. It was proclaimed that the state health care system should be changed to a public one.

Advisers to the President in the spheres of health and environment and women, family, and children were nominated and functioned in 1991–1994. They were active in public health issues, emphasizing the need to control high mortality and preserve the environment.

The first state public health report was commissioned by the President in 1992, presented by the President to the National Parliament, and pub-lished. A presidential decree prescribed preparation of the report on an annual basis. A recommendation for the administrative territories to pre-pare similar reports was issued.

In 1993, health information was declassified by the Federal Law of State Secrets. A national security concept (Concept of National Security of Russian Federation, 2000) was adopted, incorporating social security and public health issues. The bases of legislation of the Russian Federation on protection of the health of citizens were approved, including revised prin-ciples of health care. In December 1993, after a conflict among federal branches of power, a new constitution was adopted.[20]

---

[20]According to Article 41: (1) Everyone has a right to health protection and medical care. Medical care for citizens at state and municipal health care facilities is provided free of charge by means of respective budget and insurance payments and other receipts. (2) In the Russian Federation, the federal programs for population health protection and strengthen-ing are funded, measures are implemented aimed at the development of state, municipal,

During this first period, however, a broad crisis characterized by political changes, economic hardships, security issues, and the conflict in Chechnya drew the attention of individuals, the society, and the state, and public health concerns were overshadowed and reduced to health care reform. The latter emphasized the introduction of medical insurance. That shift resulted in such problems as the neglect of public health, disease prevention, and health promotion, as well as inappropriate use of health funds. Despite constitutional guarantees, a several-tier health care system has become firmly established. Drug supplies and access to expensive quality health care became a matter for public concern.

The response to public health challenges, even the depopulation threat, was inadequate. Some experts and scholars even referred to depopulation as a trait of developed societies, which Russia aspired to be. The financial crisis of August 17, 1998, exacerbated the political, economic, social, and public health crisis, and resulted in modification of the path forward.

The second period began in 2000, when Vladimir Putin was elected president. At that time, the overall crisis and depopulation were continuing.

Russia's new leadership became increasingly aware of the need to prevent depopulation, particularly in Siberia and the Far East, to ensure the survival and stability of the country. Russia's global security role (beyond issues of weapons of mass destruction), acknowledged by its membership in the Group of Eight (G8), also necessitates alleviation of public health problems.

In his first Address to the National Parliament on July 8, 2000 (Rossiyskaya Federatsiya, 2000), President Putin reviewed the most pressing issues Russia is facing, citing a forecast of population decline. In his words, in 15 years the country's population could decrease by 22 million, and the survival of the nation would be endangered if this trend were to persist. A closely related public health priority for the new administration is effective management of migration. The policy response includes instituting pronatalist and health-promoting policies and/or revising immigration policy. In any case, the role of the federal government is central as sponsor and market regulator. This is illustrated by the experience of the developed world, especially Western Europe and Japan.

In September 2001, the concept of demographic development of the Russian Federation (Government of the Russian Federation, 2001b) was promulgated by the federal government. For the first time in Russian his-

---

and private health care systems; activities are promoted that are beneficial for the strengthening of human health, the development of physical culture and sports, and ecological and sanitary–epidemiological welfare. (3) Concealment by officials of facts and circumstances, creating a threat to life and health, is sanctioned according to federal law (the Constitution of the Russian Federation, 1993).

tory, the state started to articulate the interests of society in the demographic sphere. The concept is a concise 11-page document and is not obligatory, nor does it include funding decisions or specify the optimal number and characteristics of population for the country. Three approaches to control of depopulation have been proposed, each entailing political, economic, and social costs.

The first is to promote pronatalist policies. Such policies promise long-term solutions. Analysis of the Soviet experience when additional benefits were provided to families having children suggests that such programs may encourage families to have children sooner than they would otherwise. Even if successful, these programs take a long time to show a significant effect on dependency ratios and can also lead to decreased participation by women in the workforce. Some politicians in Russia have suggested introducing a ban on abortions, recalling that such a measure was adopted in the USSR after World War II until 1955 and helped restore and then increase population numbers.

The second approach is to prevent premature mortality by means of health promotion and disease prevention. However, if this approach is to succeed, the social security system and informal safety nets, already strained in Russia, need to be strengthened to serve the increased numbers of aged with poor health that would survive.

The third approach is to promote immigration. This is a common practice in many developed countries, notably the United States. The Russian government is exploring replacement migration as a way to improve support ratios (Demin, 2002). Relevant legislation would have to be developed. However, this strategy could be ineffective and politically unacceptable because of the extraordinarily large numbers of immigrants that would be required. From 2000 to 2050, the net total number of migrants needed to maintain the size of the working-age population in Russia would be 32 million (nearly 650,000 per year), according to the United Nations forecasts. Promotion of large-scale immigration would thus require major cultural changes in Russia, including effective programs promoting tolerance and preventing xenophobia. Currently the number of resident aliens is small.

Moreover, control of illegal immigration has become one of the main tasks for law-enforcement bodies within the Federal Ministry of Interior. Many illegal immigrants are criminal offenders or are targets of criminal groups. The majority are involved in illegal commerce and do not pay taxes (Korich, 2002).

The strategic priority of the current Russian federal government is ensuring an increase in the revenues of households, controlling poverty, and protecting socially disadvantaged groups. The 2002 census is expected to provide additional information for public health policy development. Private enterprise in Russia thus far has proved to be socially irresponsible, with some minor exceptions.

Civil society started to develop in Russia in the 1990s. Since 1996, political parties have included public health issues, related mainly to the nation's health care model, in their electoral platforms. The Communist Party is the main opposition power; it attempted to impeach President Boris Yeltsin, and one of the issues put forward during the impeachment procedure was "genocide" of the nation. However, this party is responsible for the accumulation of public health problems during the Soviet period.

Only 10 percent of the population have adapted to the changed economic environment. About 20 percent believe there has been some improvement, and one-third do not accept the new reality and are ready to protest against it (Rimashevskaya, 1998b). The population continues to expect medical care to be a right of citizenship and believes in the idea of universal though not necessarily equal entitlement.

There has been strikingly little political protest, despite the considerable social costs of change. The political stability is explained by the legacy of the USSR regime, such as the absence of large inequalities and long-term poverty, the provision of welfare services, and compromised trade unions, as well as by the structural and institutional consequences of the neoliberal measures implemented, including increased unemployment, a decline in trade union membership, growth of the private sector, an increase in employment insecurity, and the opportunity to protest by voting the government out. Neoliberalism has enhanced possibilities for expressing discontent by means of "exit" strategies, which include informalization (earning money in the informal sector) and emigration, despite that fact that both are economic pathologies resulting from the implemented policies (Ellmann, 2000). Emigration, a direct impact of globalization, has led to the loss of large numbers of young, well-qualified, healthy, educated potential workers.

The World Health Organization (WHO) office (Moscow) for the Special Representative of the Director General was established in December 1998. Core funding is provided by a voluntary donation from the five Nordic countries. Among the office's tasks are assisting Russian health authorities in activities against TB and HIV/AIDS and addressing structural issues related to essential drugs (WHO, 2005). The threat of the spread of drug-resistant TB strains beyond national borders has attracted international attention, and relevant programs have been launched. The World Bank considers AIDS and TB to be major problems for Russia, and for several years has consulted with the Russian federal government on a $US 150 million project for control of these diseases.

CONCLUSIONS

Russia's public health challenge is unique, though it mirrors many global and regional public health trends in both developed and developing countries.

Historical developments in the twentieth century—including dissolution of the Russian Empire in 1917 and of the USSR in 1991; two radical transitions, to socialism in the late 1920s to 1991 and to a civilized market economy from 1991 to the present; an internal repressive regime (1929–1953); and the Great Patriotic War (1941–1945)—had great social and public health costs. The costs of recent post-Soviet changes in Russia to the population have thus far been greater than the benefits. Changes in Russia triggered by the dissolution of the USSR and the opening of the country to globalization took place without due consideration of their social and public health impacts by any of the political actors involved: the state, private business, civil society, and international players. Adaptation of the population to new social relations, as well as social, mental, somatic, and even biological aspects of human well-being, has been unsatisfactory. Until 2000, social policy in Russia was aimed at survival while demodernization and declining employment were shifting social development toward the corrosion of society due to social instability.

The availability of natural resources and an educated population and opening up to globalization processes cannot guarantee a country's integration into the global economy or its internal social stability if social security and public health are not a priority in global and national political, social, and economic changes. Social security and public health can decline very rapidly if their importance is underestimated by the ruling elite, with profound repercussions for national security, the economy, and survival at the national level and beyond, to the regional and global levels. With the decline of social security, public issues already resolved can return at a new level.

There is a need to overcome a gap between the reality and the image of post-Soviet changes in Russia among many political actors, as well as among international players. Programs based on irrelevant standards and developed for other types of society and stages and levels of development cannot be sustainable in Russia and collapse when external support and funding is exhausted.

The state will have to play a central role in breaking the vicious circle of poverty, inequality, disease, premature death, and depopulation during the next stage of post-Soviet reform. The approach to public health challenges should be changed. Not only the quantity but also the quality of population matters. Democratization, more private responsibility, and less state paternalism should be combined with strong state regulation.

Support to civil society and incentives for the private sector should be legislated, along with redistribution of revenues from exports and competitive sectors of the economy toward employment, raising the incomes of households, and social security. Social policy should move from sustaining acceptable living standards toward creating a comprehensive system for developing and educating individuals. Care for neglected children and strengthening of migration service are priorities, along with education, health care, and science.

More use of the positive opportunities provided by globalization—for example, telemedicine, the Internet, access to information—is needed. Discussion of globalization and public health issues should be expanded in Russia. A new paradigm of global health is needed among Russian public health leaders.

Public education is needed because an antiglobalist front, as well as xenophobia, is developing rapidly in Russia. The role of international players should be modified, especially in relation to the planned WTO accession of Russia. These players should pay more attention to the social and public health aspects of the policies pursued; otherwise, negative impacts will have a regional and global spillover effect. Peculiarities of public health theory and practice in Russia, both successes and failures, should be taken into account in the development of global public health policy and governance, with the participation of Russia. Adequate participation of Russia in global governance will depend on its success in the public health sphere.

A single system of global governance based on unification will require improved standards of national governance, with an emphasis on humanitarian issues, as well as the closing of gaps in governance and development among countries and prevention of the marginalization of whole countries and regions. Incentives for national and international players should be designed to ensure positive developments. International law on poverty might be among the first steps, as the historical development of social security in various nations suggests.

The political model of globalization should be amended. Trade interests should be subordinated to public health interests. Public health and globalization issues should be incorporated into intergovernmental cooperation programs between Russia and other countries.

A transnational research agenda in public health and globalization should be developed, especially addressing migration and infectious disease control. There are experts in Russia capable of participating in relevant activities within international collaborative programs. Russia possesses unique experience in the protection of its territory from extremely dangerous infections through its so-called counterplague service, and this experience could be useful for other countries. Russia could play a leading role in the prevention and control of HIV/AIDS and other infectious diseases in the Commonwealth of Independent States and Eastern Europe. Russian experts could work on the problem of bioterrorism prevention and control, as well as prevention of the spread of infectious diseases beyond national borders as a result of migration.

REFERENCES

Bezruchka S. 2000 (July 5). Globalization a health hazard. *The Guardian*. Issue No: 1007. [Online]. Available: http://www.cpa.org.au/garchve2/1007glob.html [accessed on September 12, 2005].

CIA (Central Intelligence Agency). 2001. *Long Term Demographic Trends: Reshaping the Geopolitical Landscape*. [Online]. Available: http://www.cia.gov/cia/reports/Demo_Trends_For_Web.pdf [accessed on September 12, 2005].

Concept of National Security of Russian Federation. 2000. Approved by Decree of President of Russian Federation from 17.12.1997 #1300 (in version of the Decree of President of Russian Federation from 10.01.2000 #24). Moscow. P. 23 [in Russian].

Dakhin VN. 2001. *The Contours of Globalization*. Svobodnaya mysl' (Free Thought) - XXI, #11. [in Russian].

Delyagin M. 2001 (April 11). Russia in conditions of globalization. *Nezavisimaya gazeta* (independent newspaper) [in Russian].

Demin AK. 2002. *Alcohol and the Health of the Population in Russia* 1900-2000. Moscow, RAOZ, (unidentified) 1999. [in Russian]. www.itar-tass.com.

Ellmann M. 2000. Chapter 5: The social costs and consequences of the transformation process. *Economic Survey of Europe* (2/3):125–140.

Fedotova VG. 2001 (February 21).*Russia in the Global and Domestic Realms. Today Being Similar to Others is Not Good Enough, One Must Be Better or Unique*. Nezavisimaya gazeta (Independent Newspaper). # 31 (2341), (in Russian).

Field MG. 1992. Soviet medicine before and after the fall. *Harvard Medical Alumni Bulletin*. Pp. 30–35.

Field MG, Twigg, JL, eds. 2000. *Russia's Torn Safety Nets: Health and Social Welfare during the Transition*. New York: St. Martin's Press. P. 314.

Gerasimenko NF. 1997. Health and politics. In: *Recommendations for Citizens and Non-Commercial Organizations for Defending the Health-Related Rights and Interests of the Population*. Moscow, RAOZ. Pp. 22–43. [in Russian].

Gerasimenko NF, Demin AK. 2002. *The Formation of Tobacco and Public Health Policy in Russia*. Moscow: RAOZ. P. 297.

Government of the Russian Federation. 2001a. *Government Report on the Health Status of the Russian Federation in 2000*. Moscow, Russia 2001. [in Russian].

Government of the Russian Federation. 2001b. *The Conception of Demographic Growth in the Russian Federation to 2015*. Approved on the order of the Government of the Russian Federation on September 24, 2001. N# 1270-r. P. 11. [in Russian].

IOM (Institute of Medicine). 1997. *America's Vital Interest in Global Health*. Washington, D.C.: National Academy Press.

Kargalitsky B. 2001. *Globalization and Russia*. [Online]. Available: http://www.zmag.org/sustainers/content/2001-03/12kagarlitsky.htm [accessed on September 12, 2005].

Kazan. 1998. *Social Hygiene (Medicine) and the Organization of Public Health*. Edited by Academician, Professor Yu.P. Lisitsin, Russian Academy of Medical Sciences. P. 697. [in Russian].

Kickbusch I, Buse K. 2001. Global influences and global responses: International health at the turn of the 21st century. In: Merson MH, Black RH, Mills AJ, eds. *International Public Health: Diseases, Programs, Systems, and Policies.* Gaithersburg, MD: Aspen Publishers. Pp. 701–737.

Kickbusch I, de Leeuw E. 1999. Global public health: Revisiting healthy public policy at the global level. *Health Promotion International* 14(4):285–288.

Koop CE, Pearson CE, Schwarz MR. 2000 (September). *Critical Issues in Global Health.* San Francisco, CA: Jossey-Bass. Pp. 1–504.

Korich Y. 2002. *The Hunt for Migrants.* [Online]. Aailable: www.vesti.ru [accessed on September 15, 2005]. [in Russian].

Lee K. 1999. Globalization and the need for a strong public health response. *European Journal of Public Health* 9(4)249–250.

Matveevskiy YA. *Globalization and Integration. The Russian Position.* [in Russian].

Rimashevskaya NM. 1998a (January). *Liberalism and Social Guarantees under the Conditions of Transition Economics: Russia in the First Half of the 1990s.* Second International Research Conference on Social Security, Jerusalem.

Rimashevskaya NM. 1998b. *Breaking Negative Tendencies in the Social Sphere.* Scientific-Practical Conference "Social Priorities and Mechanisms for Economic Transformation in Russia," Moscow (May 12–13). [in Russian].

Rossiyskaya Federatsiya. 2000. *A Message from the President of the Russian Federation to the Federal Assembly of the Russian Federation. The Government of Russia. The Path to Effective Statehood (On the Situation and Fundamental Aspects of the State Domestic and Foreign Policy.* Moscow, RAOZ, (unidentified) 1999. [in Russian].

Russian Federation. 2000. *Human Development Report on Globalization.* New York: United Nations Development Programme.

Shapiro J. 1995. The Russian mortality crisis and its causes. In: Aslund A, ed. *Russian Economic Reform at Risk.* London and New York: Pinter.

Shkolnikov V, Nemtsov A. 1997. The anti-alcohol campaign and variations in Russian mortality. In: Bobadilla J,Costello CA, and Mitchell F., eds. *Premature Death in the New Independent States.* Washington, D.C.: National Academy Press. Pp. 239-261.

The Constitution of the Russian Federation. 1993. Moscow.

UNECE (United Nations Economic Commission for Europe). 2000a. *Economic Survey of Europe.* Statistical Appendix. Geneva: United Nations. No. 1, P. 228.

UNECE. 2000b. *Economic Survey of Europe.* Statistical Appendix. Geneva: United Nations. No. 1, P. 230.

United Nations. 2002. *International Migration Report.* New York: United Nations. P. 2 [Online]. Available: http://www.un.org/esa/population/publications/ittmig2002/2002 ITTMIGTEXT22-11.pdf. [accessed on October 19, 2005].

WHO (World Health Organization). 2000. *The World Health Report 2000. Health Systems: Improving Performance.* Geneva, Switzerland: World Health Organization. P. 206.

WHO. 2005. *WHO: Russian Federation.* [Online]. Available: http://www.who.int/countries/rus/en/ [accessed on October 19, 2005].